GENTLE YOGA

FOR PEOPLE WITH ARTHRITIS, STROKE DAMAGE, M.S., OR PEOPLE IN WHEELCHAIRS

LORNA BELL, R.N. and
EUDORA SEYFER

Illustrations by
Nancy Neenan
Photographs by
Laura Cummings

CELESTIAL ARTS
BERKELEY, CALIFORNIA

READER, PLEASE NOTE: *Gentle Yoga* is not a replacement for conventional health care. Consult your doctor with your personal exercise and medical questions. Individuals vary, and you should not attempt to perform any exercises or practices without the consent of your physician.

Originally published independently in 1982 by Igram Press, Cedar Rapids, Iowa (ISBN 0-911119-01-9; Library of Congress Catalog Card Number 82-090745).

CELESTIAL ARTS
P.O. Box 7327
Berkeley, California 94707

Cover design by Ken Scott
Interior design by Paul Reed
Composition by Quadratype, San Francisco
Interior illustrations by Nancy Neenan
Photography by Laura Cummings

Library of Congress Cataloging-in-Publication Data

Bell, Lorna, 1942-
  Gentle yoga.

Bibliography: p.
  1. Yoga, Hatha—Therapeutic use. 2. Yoga, Hatha.
I. Seyfer, Eudora, 1925-   II. Title.
RM727.Y64B45 1987   615.8'2   86-28364
ISBN 0-89087-636-3

Manufactured in the United States of America

First Celestial Arts Printing, 1987

    4   5   —   96   95   94   93

CONTENTS

*To the students who inspired us by their
needs, YWCA, Cedar Rapids, Iowa.*

The important
thing is
this

To be able
to sacrifice
at any moment
what we are for
what we could become

—*Chas Du Bois*

I

Yoga: A Life-style For A Life-time

What is yoga and why do people with disabilities and special problems become such devoted students?

Yoga is a life-style. It's a non-competitive system for the development of human potential and is based on the concept of self-worth. Yoga develops a feeling of individuality. No matter what your physical condition, your age, your abilities, or your disabilities, yoga uses what you have, recognizes the wonder of you, and makes you better. People appreciate the fact that yoga appreciates them—just as they are.

Yoga is an ancient art which began in India before the birth of Christ. Although there are many branches of yoga, "hatha yoga" is the branch which has swept across America offering a totally different concept in physical fitness.

In Sanskrit, the word "yoga" means union; "ha,"

means sun, and "tha" means moon. Therefore "hatha yoga" means a balanced union—a system for creating the balanced well being of the total person. Yoga joins body, mind, and spirit into a balanced whole.

Yoga combines poses or postures (also known by the Sanskrit term *asanas*) with deep breathing, relaxation, a healthful diet and proper thinking. Almost at once, your body responds to the deep breathing and stretching: you feel better as yoga's cleansing action begins to rid your body of toxins. This results in a self-reinforcement. Because you feel better, the desire to continue is strong. Then as you are able to stretch a little farther and bend more easily, you set goals for improvement and the process is underway. Yoga can become addictive!

Yoga is not a huffing-puffing ordeal. It's a slow, thoughtful system of stretching and balancing. There is a pose which affects every muscle in the body, and the poses activate and stimulate circulation, digestion, elimination, the nervous system and the endocrine system. It has been said that your endocrine system is the medicine chest of the body—and yoga opens that cabinet door. Yoga is a potent natural medicine with a preventive, holistic approach.

Yoga is noted for its period of deep relaxation (Savasana) at the end of each yoga session. This calms the mind, slows the pulse, and brings the body to a state which is receptive for healing.

Yoga is *not* a religion. A yoga student can believe in any religion or in none at all. It is not magic—no snake charming or walking on nails. It has nothing to do with yogurt. Rather, yoga is a very practical system for improving life. It actually changes people, physically and mentally.

II

Yoga for Special Needs

Unlike other forms of physical exercise, yoga has something for everyone. No one is excluded.

People with chronic diseases and disabilities face *"can't"* at every turn in their lives: they *can't* play golf, *can't* play tennis, *can't* run, *can't* over-exert themselves, *can't* walk without a cane, some *can't* walk at all.

But everyone *can* do yoga. In yoga, there are no *can'ts*.

Yoga can be modified and adapted to suit the needs of everyone. And although yoga is not a "show off" sort of activity, people with disabilities often actually excel in some of the postures. An example is our model Arlene Henderson who is a wheelchair MSer. Her fabulous forward bend is an inspiration.

An explanation of yoga's relationship to four specific disabilities follows.

Yoga and Multiple Sclerosis

Multiple sclerosis, simply, means "many scars." It is the most common central nervous system disease among young adults in the United States. An estimated 500,000 Americans have M.S. and closely related disorders. The "many scars" are hardened tissue in various damaged areas of the brain and spinal cord (central nervous system). An individual's particular symptoms depend upon the location of the episodes of inflammation and resultant patches of scarring. This is why each person with multiple sclerosis has unique disabilities. These scarred or sclerosed areas receive a distorted or blocked flow of messages along the nerves to various parts of the body. These messages control all our conscious (voluntary) and unconscious (involuntary) movements. In other words, body functions become uncontrolled because the messages along the nerves are unable to get through, or go to the wrong area, due to this scarring. One of the criteria for diagnosis is evidence of involvement of two or more separate parts of the central nervous system in two or more episodes separated by a month or more. Hence the "multiple."

This disease is one of medicine's greatest enigmas. We've learned little more about the cause of M.S. than we knew in 1868 when Charcot, the French neurologist, first described it. He developed the diagnostic criteria known as Charcot's Triad: Intention tremors, slowing and scanning of speech, and vision abnormalities, especially rapid jerking of the eyeballs. These symptoms have been elaborated to include:

> paralysis
> spasticity
> incoordination
> shaking of hands

diminished bowel and bladder control
fatigue
numbness
slurred speech
staggering or balance problems
prickling sensations
pain in the trunk or legs
decreased breathing capacity
emotional unsteadiness
impotence or genital anesthesia

Symptoms vary not only from person to person, but from time to time in the individual. Its unpredictable nature renders this disease a cruel paradox. Remissions occur when the inflammation stops and the damage is partially repaired, but the repair is rarely perfect. It is this imperfect repair or scar tissue which causes some patients to have permanent symptoms. This fact, coupled with the doubt-riddled path often experienced before the diagnosis, and the peak productive years which are usually involved, leaves one with a feeling of the unfairness of it all. Emotional unsteadiness is considered a symptom, but the uncertainty of the future would strain the most balanced of psyches!

Theories regarding the cause of M.S. attribute it to (1) autoimmune mechanisms (2) infection by a slow virus (3) toxic agents or poisons (4) metabolic elements in the blood (5) trauma—the result of a wound, injury, or shock, and (6) lesions as a result of abnormal blood clotting mechanism. In most cases, the symptoms occur between ages 20 and 40.

No specific therapy is known. Spontaneous remissions make any treatment difficult to evaluate. The best medical treatment currently used is hormone therapy. Drugs such as ACTH and prednisone activate the adrenal glands to produce hormones which raise blood sugar, control inflammation, and alter the body's immune system. Patients

5

are also advised to build general resistance, avoid fatigue, and take muscle relaxants for spasms.

Vigorous physical exercise which over-heats the body may cause temporary worsening of symptoms. These usually clear up after a few hours rest or a cooling down period. Often a cool shower helps. This does not mean that it is harmful to exercise, but a more moderate activity may be advised. Emotional upsets are also responsible for temporary worsening of balance, strength, and coordination.

People with M.S. find that yoga can make amazing and unexpected changes in their lives. There are several possible explanations.

First, by directing the body to produce specific movements, yoga stimulates new patterns in the brain. Every time we introduce an unfamiliar movement, the motor cortex, that area of the brain which directs movements, is stimulated more completely and in a new way. Could it be that the more areas of the brain that are innervated—and yoga provides innumerable opportunities for new movement experience—the more efficiently developed our nervous systems become? Like the collateral circulation of a leg which takes over for a removed varicose vein, new pathways may augment a scarred central nervous system.

A second explanation may involve the endocrine system. We have long understood that the increased oxygen supply we get from physical activity improves thinking ability and heightens a general feeling of well being. Recent studies also indicate that daily yoga practice increases the concentration of certain endocrine products in the body. Increases in catacholamines, secretions of the adrenal medulla which tend to stimulate the nervous system, were evident in several studies. Histaminase, an enzyme that breaks down the histamine involved in allergic reactions and vasodilitation, was found to have increased. Hormones known as steroids were also affected. These substances have dynamic effects on M.S. patients. Stimulating them naturally through hatha yoga merits continued study.

Lastly, yoga is fun! If yoga were not interesting enough to challenge people with M.S., it would be impossible to motivate them to practice it. But because they truly enjoy yoga, they practice it and the slow stretching movements tone their muscles without increasing body temperatures while the relaxation techniques offset stress and emotional upsets.

It's no wonder that people with M.S. become such enthusiastic yoga students.

Yoga and Arthritis

It is estimated that seventeen million Americans suffer from some form of arthritis. Ranking second only to heart disease as the most widespread chronic disease in the U.S., arthritis affects one of every eleven Americans. More than 97% of people over 60 have arthritis severe enough to appear on X-rays.

"Arthritis" means inflammation of a joint, especially the joint lining. The two main types of arthritis are rheumatoid arthritis and osteoarthritis. It is important to know which type of arthritis is involved, and to have professional guidance from a physician or therapist in order to avoid compounding a problem.

Rheumatoid arthritis is a chronic disease characterized by painful swelling (often in the fingers), fatigue, stiff muscles, and joint deformity. Early immobility comes from tense muscles rather than joint damage, in the patient's efforts to avoid pain. Chronic muscle tension due to low-level long-standing stress is being considered as a factor in the cause of arthritis. This makes yoga with its emphasis on gentle movements, stretching and relaxation training a natural for the arthritic person. The student's goal should be to prevent deformity by maintaining joint movement and muscle strength. (Muscles support joints.) Isometric exercises are valuable, with the student using prolonged contraction before relaxation, and not simply "wiggling" the part. The student should be aware that the flexor muscles are predominantly strong (e.g. the muscles on the palm side of the hand) and should not be allowed to freeze in flexed positions. Opposite movements such as stretching the hand open, or turning prone to prevent hip contractures, are helpful. The use of a swimnming pool, warm bath, or whirlpool before exercising often makes bodywork less painful.

Osteoarthritis is regarded as a process of aging. It is the result of prolonged wear and tear on the joints, repeated injury, or joint abuse from obesity. It usually develops slowly with stiffness and pain, almost never with swelling or redness. Activity must be carefully monitored to avoid trauma and further wear on the joints. Again, Gentle Yoga is ideal for osteoarthritis.

The following suggestions are important for students with all forms of arthritis:

1. Balance periods of activity with rest. Avoid fatigue and prolonged sitting in one position.

2. Use range of motion exercises to prevent tendon tightening and flexion deformities.

3. Practice good body mechanics and postural alignment.

4. Learn relaxation techniques. Use them to assess muscle tension, especially in jaw, shoulders, spine and hands.

5. Avoid emotional strains which lead to stress. Try to practice yoga's positive thinking to modify problems.

6. Avoid jerking or jumping movements.

7. Observe your own body for imbalances in strength. Gradually improve tone with your corrective yoga program.

8. Keep body weight at a minimum. Overweight causes an unnecessary strain on the joints.

9. Avoid massage of a painful joint as this may cause more pain.

10. Do yoga daily.

A discussion of arthritis would not be complete without the mention of diet. Although it is a controversial subject, nutritional factors are highly suspect by many medical people in their studies of arthritis. Recent findings indicate that elimination of nightshade plants (tomatoes, potatoes, eggplant, peppers and tobacco) can benefit as many as 70% of arthritis sufferers. Sugar, caffeine, alcohol, red meat, and wheat are also possible factors. Allergies are being studied, as well as mineral imbalances, especially the relationship of calcium and phosphorus.

However, until all the facts are in, no one can go wrong by following the yoga approach of wholesome, high-nutrition foods consumed prudently.

Yoga and Stroke

Stroke, frequently referred to as a cerebral vascular accident or CVA, results from reduced blood supply to the brain. It can be due to a clot, hemorrhage, or poor circulation. The amount of function regained depends upon many factors, such as the site and extent of involvement. The permanence of damage cannot be predicted for at least six months. By the time a stroke victim is ready to study yoga, she will have been through a period of rehabilitation and will have experienced some improvement as the body repairs itself.

Stroke victims should have their doctor's approval before studying yoga and often a friend or relative is needed to help and support. If the student is receiving physical therapy, efforts should be made to reinforce and cooperate with the therapist's recommendations. In the case of hemorrhage, aneurism, or high blood pressure, the student should avoid activities which cause expansion of the blood vessels of the brain such as vigorous exercise, straining, hot whirlpool baths, and especially the reverse postures which place the brain below the level of the heart.

Yoga is especially helpful for these students as they learn to protect their joints, improve muscle strength on both sides, and develop a better sense of balance and positional awareness. A sense of independence is gained as the student assumes a responsible role in his yoga program. Postures should be chosen which preserve joint motion, stimulate circulation, and reestablish neuromuscular pathways. Frequent short periods of exercise are better than long vigorous sessions. The student should work within individual limitations and should rest if she feels dizzy, sweaty, or if the pulse becomes rapid.

Special problems of the stroke student with partial paralysis revolve around prevention of deformities. The student should understand that flexor muscles are stronger than extensor muscles. In other words, the muscles which draw the limbs toward the midline of the body (e.g. curl the fingers, point the toes) become very active and, if this unbalanced positioning is allowed to persist, muscle shortening occurs and joint changes take place. Frequently shoulders become "frozen" or "foot drop" and hand, wrist and arm contractures develop on the effected side. Because of the extended recovery time, lack of motion and inactivity compound the major problems of stroke recovery: verbal, visual, orientational, and neuromuscular. The recuperative time is often spent sitting in a chair, sitting in bed, or sitting in a wheelchair. This time spent in sitting upright contributes to hip flexion problems. Paradoxically, hip joint flexibility is necessary in normal walking, a skill which often needs to be relearned.

Yoga's system of precision alignment is a real bonus to the student who has had a stroke. The positions encourage balanced flexibility and strength. Nowhere is yoga's basic concept of balance and harmony more obvious than when dealing with the problems of the stroke student. Balance is more than not falling; it is an equanimity and accord within the individual, and between the individual and his surroundings.

Yoga and the Wheelchair Student

There are an estimated 645,000 Americans confined to wheelchairs. This is about three in every thousand people. The reasons for their confinement are many and varied: amputation of limbs, birth defects, spinal cord injuries, polio, cerebral palsy, and muscular dystrophy, as well as stroke, multiple sclerosis, and arthritis. A wheelchair provides freedom of ambulation for an individual who would otherwise be limited to a life in bed. For the unstable or easily fatigued, it opens new worlds of enrichment: shopping, trips to the theater, museums, zoo, participation in classes and meetings, and all those things which add so much to the human experience. With society's growing awareness of the need for barrier-free passage, people who use wheelchairs are less limited in their daily lives than ever before. There are wheelchairs tailored to every ability and need, adjusted to fit each body and disability. They run on arm power or electricity, can go up to 20 miles an hour, and can climb a 50 degree grade. Wheelchairs can pick you up or lay you down, even respond to a puff of air or the poke of a tongue. Many communities have them to loan for trips or special occasions. Wheelchairs can truly make life easier.

They can also make the body lazy! Always bear in mind this major principle: If *you don't use it, you lose it.* The wheelchair should be a tool, not a back brace. If the wheelchair is used to replace the legs, it must not be allowed to replace back and torso muscles also! If a student is able to use the back and abdominal muscles, she should use them. A student should sit up in the wheelchair, keeping the back away from the support as much as possible. The arms should move in all directions, not just to power the chair's wheels. Students should lift their arms overhead, twist and turn their torsos, shoot baskets, clap their hands. There is even an aerobic dance routine designed for use in a chair which can be adapted for most wheelchair people. Students in wheelchairs should try to use all the abilities they possess to the fullest. S/he should adjust to true limitations, but must not lose a physical function from disuse.

If it is possible, wheelchair students should be lifted out of their chairs to a floormat for yoga practice. Sitting on the floor is much better for muscles and joints than sitting in a chair. If the student is weak or unable to balance at first, a friend may sit back-to-back for support. The student should try to roll over, stretch the spine, crawl or creep, and do any of the postures she possibly can.

However, even sitting in a wheelchair, there are many yoga postures to be practiced. Deep breathing and relaxation are also extremely beneficial. Yoga makes wheelchair students feel like separate entities, rather than simply extensions of their wheelchairs.

III

The Miracle of Breath

Do you realize that everything you do or think or feel is reflected in your breathing?

If you're happy and relaxed, your breathing is calm and regulated. If you exercise, your breathing becomes rapid and shallow. If you're angry, nervous or depressed, your breathing becomes uneven and spasmodic. And while you sleep, your breathing is deep and rhythmic. To illustrate how closely breath is related to activity, ask a friend to spend the next thirty seconds concentrating all of his attention on some object you hold in your hand. He will probably slow his breath markedly, or even suspend it, as he concentrates.

The student who masters the science of breath can relieve tension, curb the appetite, improve digestion, lower blood pressure, slow the heartbeat, control emotions, and calm the mind. Deep breathing increases the supply of oxygen to the brain and, as a result, improves thought and creativity. It's even possible to breathe in a way that cleanses the lungs and prevents disease.

Another aspect of breathing that is helpful to the disabled student is the use of visualization with breath. Sustained deep breathing can pump oxygen-laden blood through the whole body, improving circulation in parts which cannot move and otherwise would get little oxygen. And by breathing deeply with concentration, it is possible to direct warming and healing energy into an area. This technique is discussed in the chapter on relaxation.

Pranayama

The major benefit disabled students gain from yogic breathing is the energy boost they experience. Pranayama, the name given to this branch of yoga, literally means the extension or control of our energy or life force, termed "prana." Because fatigue is a common problem for Gentle Yoga students, the potential benefits of yogic breathing alone are great enough to merit the serious study of yoga.

Most of us use only one-ninth of the total capacity of our lungs for normal breathing. This usual breath contains about 500 ml. or roughly two cups of air. This type of breathing is shallow, inefficient—and hard work to boot! By utilizing yoga breathing techniques, you can increase your capacity to oxygenate blood, as well as train and strengthen the muscles which control respiration.

Because the study of Pranayama begins with breath control, a basic understanding of the anatomy and physiology of the respiratory system is helpful.

The trunk consists of two parts: the thoracic cavity or

chest and the abdominal cavity. The lungs hang suspended in a closed cage—the thoracic cavity. They are soft and sponge-like, and have no contractile ability of their own. They expand in the vacuum created by the surrounding ribs and intercostal muscles, and the diaphragm below. This diaphragm consists of a thick muscle which forms the floor of the thoracic cavity. When it contracts, it becomes flat creating more space in the chest. This descending of the diaphragm causes surface tension, the pressure between the lungs and chest wall changes, and air rushes into the expanded lungs. It is the focus on the abdomen moving forward and enlarging, then, that first teaches the student to move his diaphragm because, as the diaphragm descends (contracts), it presses abdominal contents forward. Hence: "Inhale, ballooning out your abdomen."

Exhaling either occurs passively, at the end of a normal breath, or forcefully, requiring coordination of diaphragm, chest, and abdominal muscles. Training these muscles greatly augments their action.

Because breathing is at the very core of yoga, deep breathing is the first thing taught to beginning students. There are many yoga breathing techniques, but the following techniques provide a basis for the beginner's practice.

Rules to Remember

1. Always breathe through the nose. Yogis believe that the mouth is for eating and talking. The nose with its built-in filtering system, warms and cleans the air before it enters your lungs.

2. Persevere in your practice. Beginners get discouraged and feel they aren't doing anything. Advancement is slow but improvement is progressive.

3. Never strain or practice to exhaustion. If your

knuckles are white, you're too tense. This will be self-defeating. Work within your comfortable limits and stop if you have chest pain or side aches.

4. Try to practice in the cleanest air available. Fresh air or a well ventilated room is preferable.

5. Practice with an empty stomach.

Diaphragmatic Breathing

(Also called the abdominal breath because the focus of movement is in the forward protrusion of the abdomen.)

Technique:

1. Assume a position of rest. Beginners should practice on their backs with a book or hand on the abdomen below the waist. After this has been mastered, the student may sit erect.

2. Relax as you focus on how you are breathing. It helps to close your eyes. Inhale as you stretch the abdomen outward. Exaggerate this movement at first,

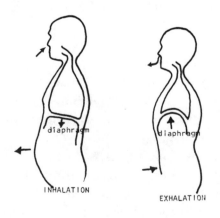

breathing through the nostrils in an even, steady manner. Beginners can observe the motion of the abdomen by watching the book or hand placed on the abdomen.

3. Follow each inhalation with an exhalation, pressing in and back with the abdominal muscles.

4. Each massive exhalation is followed by an equally great inhalation. The shoulders and upper chest should not move with the breath.

5. Concentrate on directing energy to the solar plexus, recharging and revitalizing the body.

Practice this technique until you are sure you have it right. When it feels easy and second nature, practice it sitting up, with a straight back, anytime you think of it—while riding in the car, waiting in line, when you're put on "hold" on the phone. Just be sure the air you're breathing is clean and fresh. This will reinforce your practice and energize you throughout your day. Master this technique before going on to the next.

The Complete Breath

The object of the complete breath is to saturate the lungs with as much energy or "prana" as possible. Practice this after the diaphragmatic breath has been mastered.

Technique:
1. Relax, close the eyes and become centered.

2. Inhale slowly through the nose. First, fill the abdomen, letting it balloon out. Next, stretch the ribs out as the middle chest fills. Then fill upper lungs under the sternum and shoulders.

3. Hold the breath.

4. Exhale slowly reversing the sequence in #2. Be sure to squeeze out all stale air.

5. Continue the smooth flow of one breath after another, watching for an increase in depth. As practice continues, the breath will grow steady and longer in duration. The sounds of this steady passage of air over your soft palate will create a soothing metronome, a relaxation technique in itself.

NOTE: Many books suggest a ratio of a certain number of "counts" or seconds for each section of the exercise, i.e. eight seconds, inhalation; hold for eight; exhale for sixteen. Or inhale for five, hold for five, exhale for five. As no two people are exactly alike, so no uniform number will suit all students. Work to capacity, strive to gently increase your number, and experiment with the ratio which feels comfortable to you. Then, don't be afraid to change it.

"Ha" Breath

This breath empties the lungs in a dynamic way, expelling the stale breath from deep in the lungs. This breath almost totally exchanges the stale air in your lungs for fresh, clean air. It is the stagnant air at the base of your lungs that harbors the germs which cause infection. You may want to practice this breath early in the sequence so you start your practice with clean, unpolluted air.

1. Raise the arms overhead, either from a standing or sitting position, inhaling deeply.

2. Lower the arms as you forcefully expel all the air you can through your open mouth. (This is one of the few times you use your mouth.) Make an audible hissing "HA" sound, which should last about five seconds or until all the air you have is expelled.

3. Repeat several times.

The Bellows Breath

"I haven't had a cold since I learned the Bellows Breath." This is a common statement among yoga students—and a common experience for anyone who practices the Bellows Breath daily. This technique cleanses and aereates the system, and recharges the body by rapidly pumping air in and out. All the action is in the abdomen which acts like a bellows. The passage of air reminds one of the chugging of a train's locomotive. As well as cleansing the lungs dynamically, this breathing technique promotes strength and tone of the abdomen and diaphragm. Coordination of these two muscles is a by-product. NOTE: Be sure the mouth is closed. Breathing is through the nose only. If dizziness occurs, consult a teacher for guidance. Don't "hyperventilate" by breathing rapidly through the mouth.

Technique:

1. Sit in a comfortably erect position. Be sure the spine is straight.

2. Breathe in a small amount of air through the nose, ballooning out the abdomen. Visualize clean air and energy coming into the lungs.

3. Without pausing, exhale, snapping back the abdominal muscle. This is a short, forceful expulsion of air with more emphasis on exhalation than inhalation. Visualize stale air, smoke, and waste leaving the body.

4. Immediately follow this action by a relaxed forward movement of the abdomen. This action, too, is short and small. Repeat these motions in a coordinated fashion, as rapidly as you can without loosing the rhythm. A breath per second might be a goal to achieve. Begin with five in a row, working up to three sets of fifty each.

Alternate Nostril Breathing

"Nostril dominance," or the shifting in openness of the nasal passages, is a fascinating phenomenon which has recently attracted the attention of Western researchers.

The whole nervous system of man is like a great battery. The autonomic nervous system, which is self-controlling, regulates involuntary responses such as nutritive, vascular, and reproductive functioning. It is divided into two branches: the sympathetic, which can be viewed as "positive," stimulating activity, and parasympathetic, the "negative," quieting force.

With a little practice, you can determine which of your nostrils is more open or dominant. If you moisten your wrist, and exhale the breath forcefully through the nose, one side will have more air flow. You may notice that air from the right side feels warmer. Yogis call this side "pingala," which means sun. This corresponds to the sympathetic or positive force which stimulates function. The left, called "ida," is cool like the moon and has an inhibitory effect on the body. These two forces are said to begin at the nose and intersect at six places along the spine called "chakras" and considered storage places for energy, or the battery of man.

In the healthy individual, yoga asserts, there is a rhythmic cycle of about two hours in which the nostrils alternate dominance. It is believed that prolonged breathing from the left side affects the body by inhibiting function, leaving the individual cold, tired and lethargic. Conversely, over-dominant right breathing over-works the acceleratory mechanisms, leaving the individual hot, nervous, and distraught. The flow of air in equal amounts through both nostrils is ideal.

If an alternating cyclic change of nostril dominance

maintains a healthy equilibrium in body functioning, the student can understand the importance of monitoring the nostril breathing pattern, particularly when feeling ill or tired, and using the following techniques to control the flow.

Technique

Sit in a comfortable position with back straight. Using the right hand, place the middle finger on the forehead, between the brows. The right thumb rests gently over the right nostril, and the little and ring fingers rest against the left nostril. Breathe slowly and deeply through both nostrils. As you isolate one side for breathing, the fingers will gently obstruct the other, rotating the active or open side back and forth alternately.

1. Press the right nostril closed with the thumb, inhaling steadily through the left nostril for the count of 5.

2. Pinch both nostrils closed as you hold the air in the lungs for the count of 5.

3. Lift the thumb, exhale, count of 5, through the right nostril.

4. Without a pause, inhale through the right nostril (through which you just finished exhaling), hold for 5 counts, and exhale through the left nostril.

Briefly:
- Inhale left for 5
- Hold for 5
- Exhale right for 5
- Inhale right side, 5
- Hold for 5
- Exhale left, 5

The above is one complete round. Do five rounds, breathing slowly, deeply and quietly. The effect is calming with a pleasant lightness in the sinus areas of the face. You'll see why this exercise is often recommended for insomnia and sinus problems as well as for the fatigue and nervous problems which often plague the chronically ill.

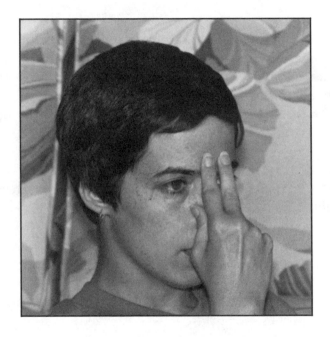

I hear
   & I forget

I see,
   & I remember

I do,
   & I understand

   —Chinese proverb

IV

The Postures

And now we come to the postures or poses.

Knowing that the needs of each student are different, we have included the directions for many postures. We suggest that you read through the chapter and choose a group from those poses which your body is able to do. Then practice your special sequence at the same time each day. Try to find a time when you will have no interruptions. Some students prefer morning practice in order to start the day with increased circulation and a feeling of well being; others like evening practice to prepare for a restful night's sleep.

Devote a reasonable amount of time to your practice. Forty-five minutes per day is ideal, but fifteen minutes daily is better than long sessions once or twice a week. Always wait an hour-and-a-half after meals. Wear comfortable, loose clothes or leotards. Most people prefer to practice with bare feet.

Use common sense in your yoga practice: read the directions carefully, move into each posture slowly with awareness, and pause at the point of your own body's maximum stretch. Hold the pose and feel your body's response to it. Then, slowly, come out of the pose and rest. Usually it is beneficial to repeat the posture two or three times.

Never hold your breath during a posture. And never strain or force your body. Stretch gently, searching for any tension that may be limiting your flexibility. Then stop at your "edge" or current limit. Always begin your practice with deep breathing and end with relaxation.

You will soon notice changes in your body. Perhaps one of the most obvious differences will be improved posture. For years, many of us have carried our heads forward of our center of gravity or spinal column. Because the head weighs ten pounds, this puts a strain on the upper neck and back. These muscles become elongated and weak. To make matters worse, the opposite muscles on the front of the chest and shoulders are strong because we use them often in daily activities. However, stretching these front muscles while contracting the upper back muscles eventually pays off in a harmonious balance of both muscle groups. Yoga students become proudly erect, not an exaggerated military straightness, but balanced and lifted with ease and grace. Even wheelchair students notice a marked improvement.

Another difference in your body may be the absence of low back pain which has become America's most common complaint. This is because most low back pain is actually caused by weak abdominal muscles, and yoga soon strengthens them.

You will, of course, become far stronger and more flexible. Keep a yoga notebook and record your progress. List your daily schedule of poses as a beginning yoga student. Soon they will seem elementary and you will add others. Your progress will amaze you.

Sample Practice Schedule

Formula	**Example**
Breathing exercises	Diaphragmatic breathing
Gentle warm-ups	Neck rolls
	Shoulder shrugs
	Chest expander
Forward stretch	Forward bend
Backward stretch	Cobra
Lateral stretch	Atlas
Spinal twist	Seated twist
Hip and thigh stretch	Butterfly
Balance posture	Tree
Reverse posture	Baby headstand
Special emphasis (postures chosen for specific individual needs)	See yoga therapy index

Relaxation

Table of Postures

Although many important postures have not been included, the following postures have been class-tested by Gentle Yoga students.

Yoga Therapy Index of Postures

Asthma	Diaphragmatic breathing; Fish
Abdominal cramps, nausea	Fish; Bridge
Abdominal toning	Twist; Ceiling-walk; Mod. Sit-ups (Curl; Crunch)
Backache, acute (during)	Child; T-twist; Knee-hug; Standing forward bend; Plough
Backache, chronic (to strengthen)	Cobra; Half locust; Boat; Triangle II; Cats
Bursitis, shoulder tightness	Shoulder stretch; Warrior; Chest expander
Colds, sore throat	Lion; Shoulderstand
Concentration, mental clarity	Deep breathing; Relaxation and Visualization techniques; Shoulderstand; Baby headstand; Plough; Tree
Constipation	Abdominal lift; Knee hug; Shoulderstand; Perineal exercise
Eyestrain, vision problems	Eye Exercises
Fatigue	All breathing exercises; Shoulderstand; Plough; Stick against a wall; Relaxation techniques
Flabby/weak upper arms	Modified push-ups; Dips; Wheelchair push-up; Lift
Foot drop; ankle weakness	Foot flap; Ankle rotation; Tree; Triangles; "Ha" squat
Gas pains	Knee hug; Abdominal lift; Forward bends

Hamstring tightness	Plough; Dog; Leg stretches
Hand/finger stiffness	Hand extensor muscle lift; Hand warmer; Shaking out
Hangover headache	Plough
Hemorrhoids	Baby headstand; Shoulderstand; Shoulderstand with a wall; Perineal exercise
Hip/thigh joint tightness	Bow; Bridge; Cobra; Butterfly; Frog; "Ha" squat
Postural alignment	Tree; Tree on the floor; Chest expander
Round shoulders/ Dowager's hump	Chest expander; Bow; Camel; Warrior
Sciatica	Frog; Half lotus; Twist
Shallow breathing	Fish; All breathing exercises
Sinus congestion	Baby headstand; Shoulderstand; Alternate nostril breathing
Stiff neck	Neck rolls; Shoulder shrugs; Twist
Swayback	Locust; Bridge; Lift; Forward bend; All abdominal toning exercises
Throat firming, toning	Cobra; Neck rolls; Camel; Lion
Thyroid imbalances	Shoulderstand; Plough; Baby headstand
Urinary incontinence	Perineal exercises
Varicose veins	Shoulderstand; Stick using a wall
Waist trimmer	Twists; Atlas; Triangle II; All abdominal toners

Chest Expander

BENEFITS: Many names are used for this pose, but all teachers agree it is unexcelled for postural alignment, warming up, and unkinking the chest, shoulders, spine and legs. This is especially recommended for the student with round or tight shoulders, hump back, swayback, or other back problems.

TECHNIQUE: Stand straight and relaxed. Feet should be parallel and a few inches apart. Open the arms as you breathe in deeply. (#1) Bring palms together behind you and interlace fingers, keeping your arms as straight as you can. Feel the shoulders stretching down and back. (#2) Slowly bend your head back and, if it feels right, arch back gently. Push downward with the clasped hands. (#3) Slowly and gently return to erect position, begin exhaling, and bend forward from the hips. Keep intensive stretch and resistance between the arms, and lift clasped hands as far from the back as possible. Hold (#4) Then straighten to an upright position with the next inhale breath. Release the hands, relax the neck and shoulders and observe. You should feel balanced, straighter, and you may feel tension being released from the arms and shoulders.

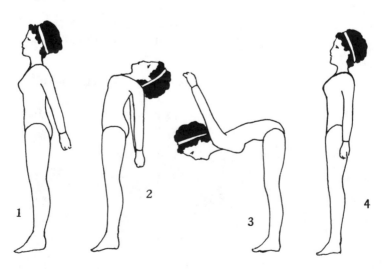

Forward Bend

BENEFITS: This pose is so vital for spinal flexibility that it is one of the criteria for setting minimum flexibility standards in the universally used Krause-Weber tests. It promotes suppleness of the spine, the abdominal organs are toned, and abdominal fat and bloating are decreased. The backs of the legs get an intense stretch.

TECHNIQUE: Stand straight. Raise the arms with a deep inhale. Stretch well, as the raised arms reach forward and then down, leading the body in its descent. The back should not be allowed to round, but should remain slightly concave (#2). This halfway point is enough for the student with spinal disc problems. With knees straight, let your body fall forward from the hips. Relax the neck, arms, and shoulders as you hang loosely at your tight stretch. If your fingers touch the floor, that's great, but don't use this as a goal and push yourself. Remain in the stretch for several seconds and then straighten. Loosely position the waist, trunk, shoulders, neck, and head upon the hips in the erect beginning position. NOTE: If the abdomen is pulled up and lifted toward the spine, you will increase your stretch considerably.

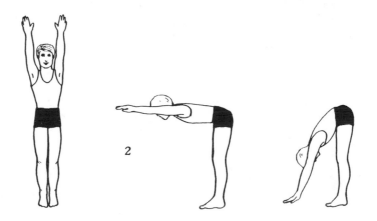

2

Triangle I Pose

BENEFITS: Torso flexibility, elongation of the spine, and stronger, more flexible feet, ankles, knees and legs.

TECHNIQUE: Place the feet about three feet apart (or about the length of one of your legs) with the right foot turned out to 90 degrees, and the left foot turned 30 degrees. The right heel should line up with the middle of the left foot.

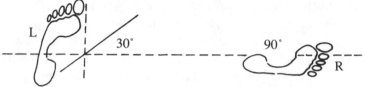

Inhale as you stretch arms out from shoulders (#1). Bend at the hips as you stretch the torso sideways. Be sure not to bend forward, but to the side. Rest the right arm on the shin where it falls, and extend the other vertically toward the ceiling. (#2) Both knees should remain straight. Hold for several breaths. Then release, rest, and reverse.

A wall provides the ideal way for the unsteady student to gain precision without falling. It also serves as a reminder to keep the back straight: the spine, hips, and shoulders should all touch the wall.

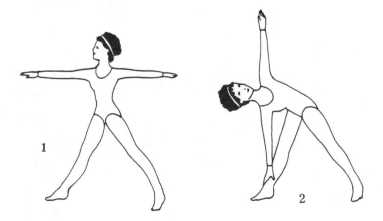

Triangle II Pose (Twisting Triangle)

BENEFITS: Same as Triangle I plus added flexibility in the hips. The torquing motion is great for a tired back as well as the spinal nerves.

TECHNIQUE: Stand as in Triangle I, feet placement at 30 and 90 degrees, and arms out at shoulder height. Inhale and rotate the upper body around in a good twist. Then stretch out and elongate spine, bend forward and rest the opposite hand on the extended leg. The free arm is extended ceilingward, and the face is turned toward it so you can see your thumb. Breathe as you hold the pose. If you have difficulty with balance, check your knees. They must be straight with knees pulled up

Revolve out of the pose slowly, rest, and observe. Then do other side.

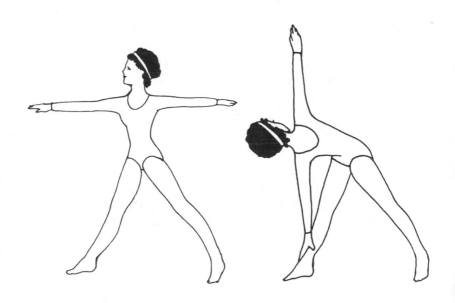

"Ha" Squat

BENEFITS: This asana is an excellent one with which to begin your yoga practice. It warms the body with an invigorating stretch, expels stale air from the lower lobes of the lungs, and stretches and opens the hip joints. A vigorous stretch is felt along the backs of the legs, particularly if the student is able to keep his heels flat on the floor. This pose strengthens and stretches the Achilles tendons, and strengthens the muscles in the fronts of the legs. Especially helpful for the student with shin splints or the MSer with "foot drop." It also relieves tension in the lower back. If necessary, the student can lightly grasp a chair back or door knob for balance.

TECHNIQUE: Stand with feet placed under hips, arms high. Inhale as you stretch the entire body, elongating through the fingertips to the toes. (#1) Stuff the body with fresh air. Then as you squat (#2) blow all the stale air forcefully out of your mouth. Take plenty of time for this. Some students will be able to keep their heels flat on the floor. By widening the distance between the feet, the stretch is made easier, while bringing the feet closer increases the challenge. Choose a variation to challenge your body.

This is an enjoyable asana to practice with another person (#3). Care must be taken not to compete. Placement of feet must be based on individual limits. Exhale as you squat. Keep the heels down. If you need to increase your stretch, back away from your partner a bit. Hold and stretch without leaning back. Inhale as you stand. Rest, then repeat.

Note: Occasionally a student is so balanced that s/he expends almost no effort in this pose, even with the feet close together. Since we must all work at our full capability, the asana can be adapted by elevating the front of the foot on a folded mat or small book.

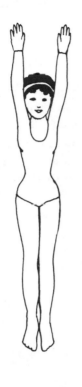

1

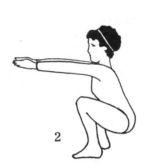

2

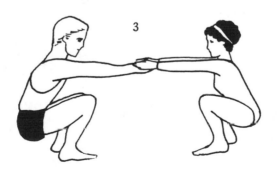

3

Tree

BENEFITS: Helps improve posture and balance. Strengthens knees, ankles and feet. As in any balance pose, concentration and an awareness of body/mind inter-relatedness are by-products.

TECHNIQUE: Stand erect, focusing your eyes on a stationary point. Bearing your weight on one leg, straighten its knee by lifting the kneecap with a tightening of the thigh muscle. Raise the other leg, positioning the sole of the foot as high as you can wedge it on the inner thigh of the standing leg (#1). Slowly raise arms. (If leg slips, try placing it upon the standing thigh, sole up as in #2.) Keep your eyes fixed on your focus point. To steady yourself, imagine a line between focus point and your eyes. Hold as long as you can. The knee and thighs are "active" and working hard, but the face and breath should remain soft and "passive." Reverse sides. Devote a little more time to your weaker side.

NOTE: Beginners may place one hand on wall for support (#3).

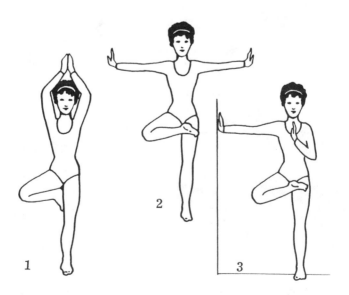

The Seated Poses

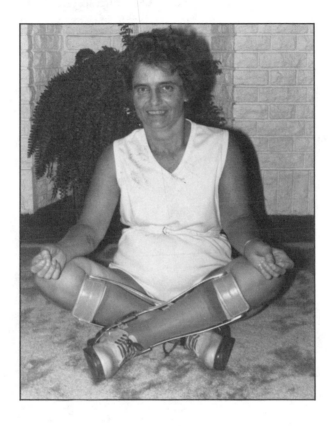

BENEFITS: These poses were originally designed to provide a straight-backed effortless sitting position from which to deep breathe, rest and meditate. However they provide much more for us today. Since we usually sit in chairs, we do not often experience the stretches upon the joints that more primitive cultures do as they sit to talk, eat, or rest. These poses provide unique ways of stretching the feet, knees and hips. Tight tendons and muscles become more elastic and supple as the poses are practiced regularly. Find the pose that is a good, comfortable stretch for you, and advance as you become more limber.

A good beginner's pose is the Tailor Seat (#1) with ankles crossed Indian fashion. Butterfly (#2) also provides a great inner thigh stretch and tones the perineum so effectively that it is recommended in natural childbirth classes. Care must be taken not to force the stretch, but gentle pressure on the knees will encourage flexibility. Students who practice this regularly usually see improvement in two months. Those students who find Butterfly (#2) easy will usually find Frog (#3) difficult as it involves the opposite way of moving the hip joint. The pose which is easy probably isn't needed as much as the one which is tight. Students who have tightness in Frog need to stretch one leg at a time, while gently supporting most of the body weight with the hands.

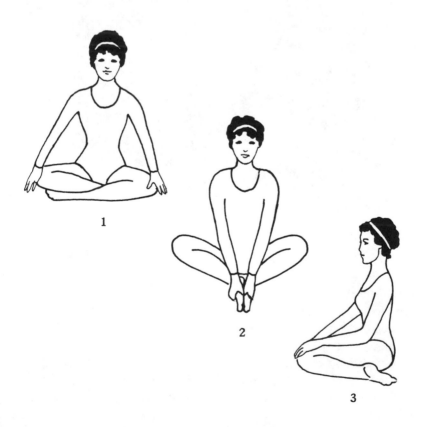

1

2

3

Hero pose (#4) presses the body weight over the bones of the feet. Feet are the farthest from the heart and tend to show signs of stiffness and age first. If sitting upon the feet is painful, place a pillow between the feet under the hips. Half-lotus (#5) is achieved by folding the heel in the perineum, and folding the opposite foot upon the thigh. Knees should be equal distance from the floor, spine erect and relaxed. Most students habitually place their "favorite" leg on top, but both sides should be given equal stretch. Full Lotus (#6) is the advanced version. The lower leg is flexed with the foot placed sole upon the opposite thigh, high into the pelvis. The other leg is flexed, lifted upward, and brought to rest on the thigh of the opposite leg. This pose has a profound effect on the circulation, sending blood which would ordinarily go to the legs to the lower spine and abdominal organs. These poses should be approached without competitiveness, and used as tools to show us where we are tight or loose, strong or weak. They are especially suitable with deep breathing, and can become a slenderizing replacement for the chair.

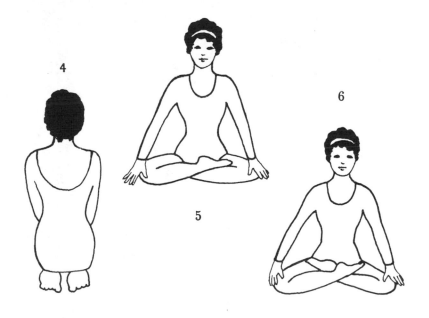

Head-To-Knee Pose

BENEFITS: This pose stretches the hamstring muscles at the backs of the legs. The forward massaging action on the abdomen tones the liver and spleen and activates the kidneys. It increases circulation in the spine and relieves low backaches.

TECHNIQUE: Sit erectly and extend one leg, pressing the back of the knee to the floor. The other leg is folded at the knee and placed at a wide angle, heel in the perineum. With an inhale breath, the arms lead the upper body in a great upward, then outward, then downward stretch. The name "head-to-knee" is really misleading: it gives the student a goal, but the student should observe where his tightness occurs and work within this stretch. Few beginning students actually fold the upper body to the head-to-knee position. It is more important to keep the back straight and enjoy the movement than to feel success or failure about distance. Hold the stretch, breathe into it, and lead the body out of the pose with the arms. Inhale as you stretch out and up and lower the arms with the exhaled breath. Rest, enjoy the after effects, and regulate the breath before testing the other side.

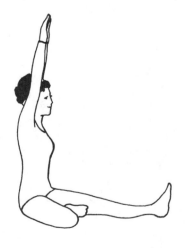
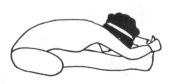

Full Forward Bend

BENEFITS: The back of the entire body receives an intense stretch. The spine becomes more elastic and a massage is given to the abdominal organs which explains its therapeutic effect on constipation.

TECHNIQUE: Sit erect, tipping the pelvis forward toward the thighs. With the legs extended, straighten the knees and "square off" the feet so that the soles are perpendicular to the legs. Inhale, opening the chest with an arm raise; exhale as you stretch outward, then downward. It is more important to keep a straight back than to round the back and bring the head closer to the floor. Relax in the stretch and allow your muscles to grow soft as you experiment with your tightness. If you move to the point of pain, you can hurt yourself. Don't strain. Spend as much time in the pose as you like. Breathe softly and notice the calming effect after you come up.

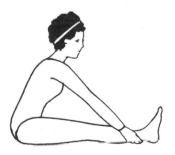

The Lift

BENEFITS: This pose counter-balances the forward bending poses. Because it works the arm muscles gently, it is a good beginning pose for women. And because it requires suppleness in the shoulder joints, it is a good pose for men. It also strengthens the wrists, ankles, legs, buttocks and back.

TECHNIQUE: Sit with legs extended and place arms behind you, fingers pointing backward. With an inhale breath, press the feet flat and lift the hips to an inclined plane. Let the head hang back, and take care to squeeze and press the buttocks high. The legs should not be allowed to roll out. Hold for a breath or two. Then simply sit down with an exhalation.

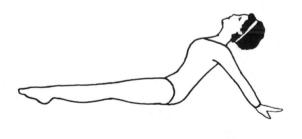

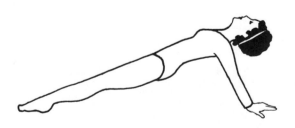

Arrow Balance

BENEFITS: This pose has much to offer the beginner as well as the more practiced student. It strengthens the abdominal muscles, the muscles in the low back, the hip muscles, and the "quads" in the fronts of the thighs. The intestines, gallbladder, liver and spleen are also rejuvenated, both by direct pressure and by the increase of their blood supply. Even the neck gets a good workout as it must work against gravity to hold the head in line. This pose also teaches balance and coordination. Many MS and stroke beginners have a distorted sense of where their bodies are in relation to space. When asked to lie on their backs with feet and hands equal-distance apart, they will be asymmetrical. Awareness and a reacquaintance with positioning are part of what we mean by balance.

TECHNIQUE: Sit on the sitting bones with back straight and knees pulled to chest. Wrap arms around shins as you shift weight to the seat and bring one or both feet slightly off the floor. (#1) Play with this balance as you experience and adjust. The breath must not be held as this makes the abdomen rigid, preventing the stimulation of the internal organs.

The following aids and variations may be used to suit various levels of ability:

A folded beach towel or blanket is helpful for the student with a prominent tail-bone. This is often the case with the slim or sedentary student, or those with diminished muscle tone in the hips.

Bringing one foot to the floor and extending the other is a gentle variation of the pose (#2). Pressing the feet to a wall (#3) is ideal for the student with weak thighs. It works the abdomen dynamically. Adjust the hips so that the feet are face high, and considerable pressure is felt between the soles and the wall.

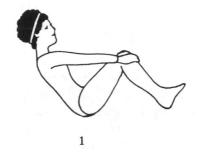

3

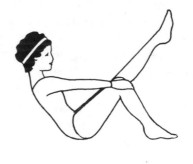

2

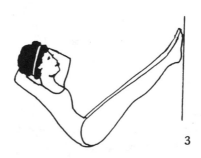

1

Spinal Twist

BENEFITS: Rotating the spinal column imparts a gentle but dynamic stretch to the intervertebral spaces and surrounding nerves. A pleasant stretch and massage are felt in the hips, waist, abdomen, and internal organs. Circulation is enhanced around the kidneys and intestines. It is not uncommon to hear a popping sound as the spine adjusts its alignment. "Ahhh!" is often heard with this pose. The twist is also an aid in reducing abdominal fat and slimming the waistline.

TECHNIQUE: Sit erect, legs extended, with your weight directly over your sitting bones. Fold the left leg. Cross your right foot over the outside of the left thigh. The outer side of the right ankle should be touching the outside of the left thigh about midpoint. Inhale, and as you exhale, rotate the trunk 90 degrees to the right keeping the shoulders level. Bring the left arm alongside the outer side of the upraised right knee. Using the left arm as a lever, grasp either the left knee or the instep of the right foot. Stretch the right arm up, around and back, placing the palm on the floor behind the seat. Turn the head over the right shoulder as you twist the upper spine. Hold, breathing shallowly. Release and repeat on the other side.

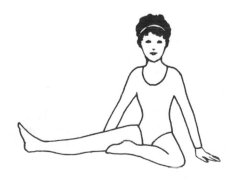
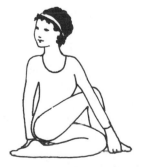

The Pose Of The Child

BENEFITS: This is a classic resting pose: a position in which to recover energy when one is tired without stopping practice. With the legs slightly parted, abdominal breathing adds to the renewal benefits. It is also the position of choice when a cramp or pain is felt in the low back. Many asanas, especially the back-arching ones, will leave the back "complaining." The stretching out of the muscles along the rounded spine affords pleasant relief.

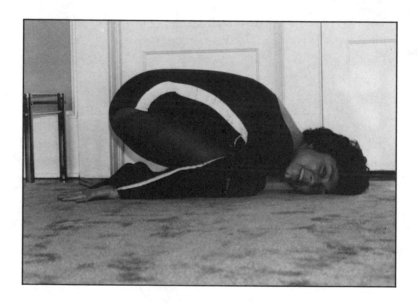

TECHNIQUE: Kneel on the mat on your shins. Stretch the upper body forward and rest the forehead on the mat. Place the arms on the floor beside the legs and relax. Breathe deeply. Turn face to one side and rest on cheek if you like.

NOTE: If it is uncomfortable to sit on the heels, place a small cushion or towel under the hips. If a large abdomen makes this asana restrictive, make a space for abdominal breathing by parting the knees.

Baby Headstand

BENEFITS: Because this pose looks unfamiliar to new students, they are usually wary of it. They soon learn it can be accomplished with relative ease and they enjoy the benefits of reversing the force of gravity: when the head is below the level of the heart, the brain is flushed with fresh blood, the pituitary and thyroid glands in the head and neck are stimulated, and coordination between the three points of balance introduces new movement patterns which develop the motor cortex of the brain.

TECHNIQUE: From the pose of the child, sitting on the heels, raise buttocks up and roll weight toward the crown of the head. The hands can be placed beneath the shoulders, near the ears, as the neck is gently stretched. (1) Distribute weight between the hands, knees and head. (2) Adjust knees until they are directly beneath the hips. Lift lower legs and grasp the shins so the body resembles the letter "n." (3) Hold as long as is comfortable, then fold into child and rest. Notice the feeling of equilibrium and increased circulation in the face.

NOTE: Not for the student with high blood pressure or glaucoma.

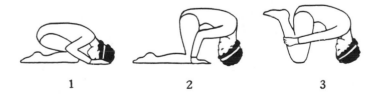

1   2   3

Table

BENEFITS: For the healthy, adept student, this pose is used as a transitional pose, one which facilitates movement from one pose to the other. But for the wheelchair student, this asana is of major importance.

Many wheelchair students begin using a wheelchair for safety and convenience. Their legs may no longer be reliable, or they may be too slow to walk in public. A wheelchair allows them the freedom of getting around. However, if special attention is not given to the abdomen, trunk, and back, the wheelchair will act as a brace, supporting the upper body like a prop. Then the muscles which hold the body erect will atrophy.

Therefore, these muscles deserve special attention. Remember, IF YOU DON'T USE IT, YOU LOSE IT! The table position requires the student to straighten the spine between the shoulders and hips, creating strength and equilibrium between the four extremities and the trunk.

TECHNIQUE: From a prone position, place the hands directly beneath the shoulders, straighten the arms, and push the hips up and back, directly over the knees. The back should be parallel to the floor, and arms and legs are placed like table legs. At first, this may be a balancing act in itself, and a helper may be needed to stabilize placement. When the pose is steady, the following cat poses will provide a continuing challenge.

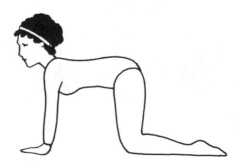

The Cat Stretch

BENEFITS: There are several variations of the cat pose. All begin from the basic "table" position and all stretch and strengthen the spine and firm the legs and buttocks.

1) CAT: CONCAVE/CONVEX

TECHNIQUE: This cat stretch vacillates between "swayback" and "humpback," using the head, and of course, the breath. With the exhaled breath, the head hangs down stretching the muscles along the back. With the inhalation, the head is raised and the waist sags down toward the floor. This pose is especially good for the student in need of gentle back strengthening.

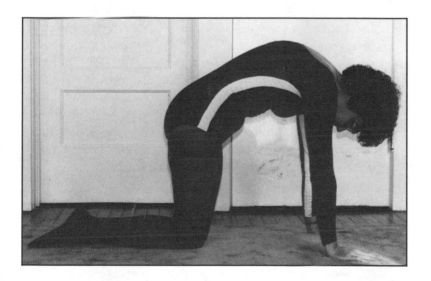

2) CAT: LATERAL STRETCH

TECHNIQUE: From "table," exhale as you turn laterally, looking over your shoulder, creating a spinal curve like the letter
"C." This compresses the organs and nerves on the inside of
the curve, while stretching the opposite side. From above, the
spine should look crescent shaped. Picture a cat looking at his
tail. Inhale as you slowly return your face to center, and exhale
as you look over the other shoulder, stretching well. Care must
be taken not to "wag" the tail; keep the hips directly over the
knees. Repeat several times, moving slowly and visualizing the
organs and spine getting a healthful toning.

3) CAT: LEG STRETCH

TECHNIQUE: This pose also begins in "table" stance, and both
hands are placed beneath the shoulders. With an inhale breath,
one leg is lifted back and up, simultaneously stretching the chin
upward, creating an arc. Smoothly, with the exhalation, the
knee is bent and brought forward to the chest. The head is
curled under, in an effort to touch the knee to the nose. (It's not
necessary to touch; the effort rounds the spine, which is important.) Flow smoothly from the arc to the curl, with breath as
your metronome. Be sure to keep the pelvis parallel to the floor
so the movement is felt in the spine, not the hip. Reverse sides
before you grow tired, working both sides equally.

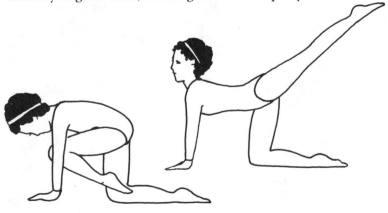

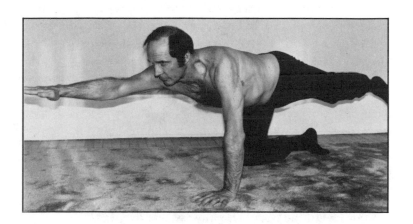

4) CAT: BALANCE

BENEFITS: Like crawling, this pose develops mental and physical coordination, and exposes the motor cortex of the brain to new movement opportunities. The extension with holding against gravity of the extremities strengthens the back as well as the limbs.

TECHNIQUE: From "table," focus the eyes upon a spot at eye level, inhale, lift and extend opposite hand and leg. Adjust weight-bearing between the supporting hand and knee/leg. The breath and face should remain soft and free of tension. Try to save enough energy to move back to "table" with grace and control. Rest, and reverse sides. It is helpful to hold the pose for a given number of breaths, rather than seconds, as the breath is often held with concentration unless there is a conscious effort not to do so. Do several before resting.

NOTE: Schoitz Hospital in Waterloo, Iowa, an institution which specializes in treating neurological patients, teaches this exercise to MSers.

5) CAT: LEG LIFT

BENEFITS: Like the other "cat" poses, this pose begins from "table" position. The other "cats," however, deal with spinal strength and flexibility. This one benefits, almost exclusively, the hip and buttock muscles, isolating them for the responsibility of lifting and extending the heavy leg, against the effects of gravity. To maximize, do slowly. This pose is intensely vigorous . . . . and intensely beneficial. Procede with awareness. Only you can decide if it is too exhausting for you. Allow plenty of recuperative deep breathing to replenish your energy.

TECHNIQUE: From "table" position, raise one bent leg so that it is level with the back. The knee is bent at a 45 degree angle, and, if placement is correct, the lower leg will be hidden from your view by the thigh. The impulse here is usually to drop the knee from this height more toward the floor, but elevating the knee is important for maximum effects. Then, accompanied by an inhalation breath, simply extend the lower leg out to the side. The extended leg should be parallel to the floor. Fold as you exhale, and continue movement with slow breathing. Then reverse sides.

NOTE: It is advisable to follow this with a forward bending stretch, to minimize soreness tomorrow.

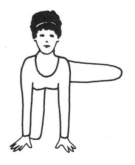 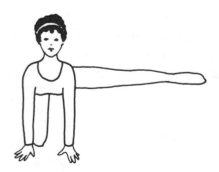

Lean Back

BENEFITS: This controlled, gradual closing of the angle between the body and lower legs is accomplished by work of the quadriceps or thigh muscles. Therefore this asana is of a strengthening or toning nature. The thighs must lengthen, but still remain contracted, as the weight of the upper body and gravity are borne in various degrees of descent. Students with thigh problems should bear in mind that there are four separate muscles in the quadriceps, and a weakness in one or two of this group does not merit ignoring the others. This asana is safe . . . you need not fear falling, you just sit!

TECHNIQUE: Kneel on a soft rug or mat. Keeping your body straight from the knees through thighs and buttocks to head, gently lean back at an inclined plane. Breathe and hold, exploring the point where quivering begins, hold for a moment, then come back to the erect position. Care should be taken not to bend at the hips.

For the student with erratic control, a rope or belt can be looped over a chest-high bar or doorknob, and adjustments can be made gradually, allowing the arms to take more or less of the weight, as is necessary.

NOTE: If this position hurts your knees don't do it! Remember, every pose is not for every body. (Knee people invariably know who they are.)

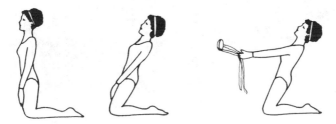

The Dog

BENEFITS: This pose is aptly named for the movements instinctively used by most dogs to awaken stiff bodies after sleeping. It is an effective way to stretch the spinal column, open and release the shoulders, and lengthen the stubborn muscles along the backs of the legs. These muscles, called the hamstrings, require persistent stretching by both sedentary people—who have short hamstrings from inactivity—and by athletes whose muscles are short and dense from repeating the same vigorous movements.

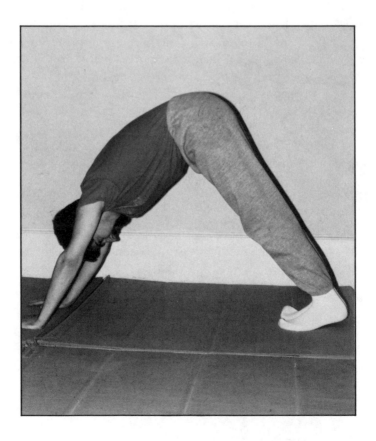

TECHNIQUE: Begin from "table" with all fours placed beneath shoulders and hips. Tuck toes under, and, on an exhale breath, straighten knees, and tip pelvis toward the ceiling. Exaggerate this stretch at first, visualizing the tail bone pointed straight at the ceiling. This permits all the stretch to be directed into the legs, rather than diffusing it throughout the small back muscles. Push with the palms, which opens the rib cage, and give yourself a moment to adjust to the increased blood flow. Breathe evenly as you relax the shoulders away from the neck. Roll high on tiptoe, then gently lower the heels toward the floor. Maintain active stretching of the pelvis, bringing the hip bones as close to the thighs as possible. Hold for three good breaths, and fold into child pose to rest.

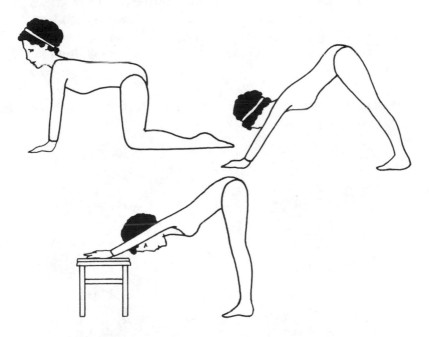

NOTE: If the student feels pain in the hamstrings, or the knees are shaky, the position can be modified by placing the hands on the seat of a stabilized chair, or on a wall, chest high. As placement is adjusted with increased flexibility, be sure to continue alignment of spine and pelvic rotation.

Camel

BENEFITS: This pose is especially beneficial for the student who has a tendency toward round shoulders. The weight of the head, at least ten pounds, augments the toning and flexibility factors of this backward bending pose. As the muscles of the upper back contract to maintain the pose, the muscles across the front of the chest are stretched and lengthened, improving circulation as well as tone and alignment. It aids in deep breathing, firms the abdomen and waist, tones the neck and throat.

TECHNIQUE: Kneel, with legs about six inches apart. Sitting on heels, lower shoulders and lift chest erect. Place hands behind feet, lean back on arms, and allow head to drop back loosely as you arch your back. (#1) From position #1, if you are in no discomfort, raise hips from heels toward ceiling. Hold for a moment, then relax. (#2)

NOTE: Not every pose is for every body. If this stretch hurts your knees, avoid it!

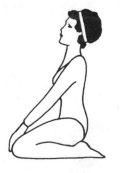 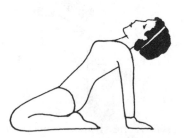

1

With body erect over knees, (3) inhale and lift one arm in an intense stretch that mimicks the swimming back stroke. Place the hand on the heel, press the pelvis forward, and drop the head, as you reach, stretch, and place the remaining hand on the other heel. Push the front of the body forward until you feel the weight of the body move from the hands and heels to over the knees. The space within the back, arms and head should form a square box. Hold, arching gently for several breaths, then recover by coordinating an exhale breath with the return of an arm to the thigh. Most students lift the head at this time. Then the other arm with the next exhale. Follow this movement immediately with a few moments in the pose of the child . . . . And enjoy the tremendous surge of warm energy surrounding your spine.

NOTE: Beginners usually have a hard time finding their feet, especially at first. This problem can be avoided by having someone support the head, or by tucking the toes under, giving the heels a higher, easier-to-reach placement. This is just a tool to teach your body spacial relationship. Later, lower the heels as pictured.

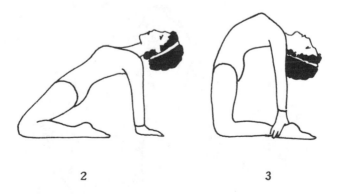

2   3

Atlas

BENEFITS: Some call this the thunderbolt posture. It limbers and slims the waistline and ribs, increases spinal flexibility, strengthens back and legs. Also gives a gentle stretch to the top of the foot and ankle.

TECHNIQUE: Sit on your "sitting" bones, both hips on the floor and feet to one side. Position the hands behind the head. With an inhale breath, lift the hips up, simultaneously raising the arms to an arc. Exhale as the hips are lowered to the opposite side. The next inhalation is accompanied by lifting up again, and lowering to the opposite side with an exhalation. Notice how the breath and upward stretching of the arms aid in raising the hips. Visualize the spine, the spinal nerves, the organs within the trunk receiving a healthy massage.

VARIATION: The wheelchair student, as well as the student sitting on the floor, can adapt the following modification. Placement of the feet is to one side, but instead of raising up, the hips remain fixed as the trunk is laterally stretched, with an elbow-toward-hips effort. As always, the inhalation takes place during the stretch upward, and exhalation with the fold. Reverse hips to the other side of the feet, and repeat. Practiced regularly, flexibility benefits are rapidly apparent.

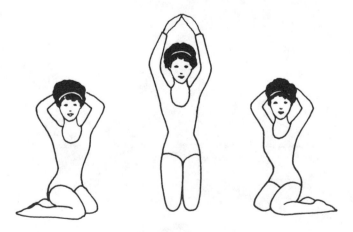

Lion

BENEFITS: The tongue is a highly vascular organ, composed of three arteries, four nerves, and numerous glands. It is important in both eating and speech, yet gets very little attention via exercise. This pose stretches the tongue by protruding it forward, and the entire organ and surrounding area are bathed in fresh, healing blood. Have you ever noticed that when you have a sore throat, you limit movement, speech, even swallowing? This inactivity contributes to the stagnation of circulation which perpetuates it. The lion does just the reverse: the tongue, neck, face and throat are flooded with blood.

TECHNIQUE: Usually this pose is done while kneeling, but can serve well from any position. A deep breath is taken in as the body is stretched upward. As a prolonged exhale brcath is expelled, widen eyes, extend tongue, and push the body forward. Stick out your tongue with intensity. Hold the extreme position for a count of ten, or until you need to inhale. Slowly withdraw the tongue as you settle back and observe. Repeat three times, unless you have a sore throat, in which case you do it six times.

In the beginning, all the attention should be on protruding the tongue. Later, you can accompany the effort with stiffening of the fingers, widening eyes, mimicking the fierceness of a lion.

NOTE: May cause gagging if practiced on a full stomach.

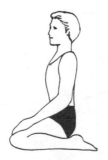 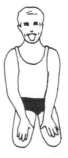

Cobra

BENEFITS: Cobra tones the entire back, expands the rib cage, stretches the front of the chest and abdomen, firms the throat, and bathes the pelvis and low back with a fresh supply of blood. The controlled backward bending brings an exhilarating supply of energy to the spine and promotes better mobility and circulation.

TECHNIQUE: Lie face down, resting brow on the mat. Stretch the body long as you firm the buttocks and bring feet snugly together. Place the palms under the shoulders and slowly begin curling the upper body as you raise the brow, nose, chin, shoulders and chest sequentially with an inhale breath. The pelvis should remain on the floor, and the shoulders should be relaxed and low. Do not push with the arms; let the spine lift as much as possible. Stop at the maximum point of stretch. Breathe. This is your limit. Respect it, but be ready to extend it as you grow with practice. Slowly uncurl as the hips, waist, ribs, chest, chin, nose, and brow smoothly descend with grace and control. Relax. Rest and enjoy the feelings of energy which are the rewards of this pose.

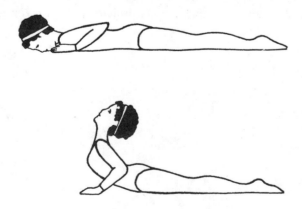

Boat

BENEFITS: Boat treats the entire posterior surface of the body to a gentle toning isometric movement as it resists gravity. This can be a beginner's pose if done slowly for one or two breaths; if held for many breaths, the effects are magnified. The front of the body—the abdomen, chest and thighs—get a refreshing stretch.

TECHNIQUE: Lie prone, stretching out long. Inhale as you arch upward, raising head and legs off the floor. Squeeze the buttocks together to protect the lower back. Arms and legs are kept straight and close together. Slowly release and relax. If cramping develops in the lower back, do child pose (page 48) to stretch it out.

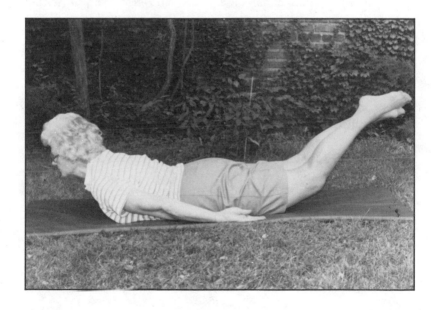

Locust

BENEFITS: This posture tones and strengthens the muscles of the lower back and buttocks, and the backs of the upper legs. It also increases circulation around the kidneys. Done regularly, this pose helps eliminate low backache and postural problems such as swayback.

TECHNIQUE: Lie face down on a mat. Bring your arms beneath your body, forming a protective "v" with the wrists together, hands interlocked forming a fist, thumbs down. Keep the toes pointed and the inner surfaces of the legs together. Rest the chin on the floor. Tighten the muscles across the small of the back, inhale and raise one leg. Hold the leg extended and as straight as possible. Feel your weight evenly distributed through your chin, arms, both hips, and passive leg. Hold for 5–10 counts, then exhale leg down and rest. Repeat with opposite leg.

#2 is for the student with weak low back muscles, or the student with a large abdomen. The pelvis is elevated in a knee-chest position.

#3 is called Full Locust, a very vigorous pose. Both legs are elevated at the same time. This should not be attempted until the single leg locust is proficient. Remember, advancement is always step by step, with regular practice.

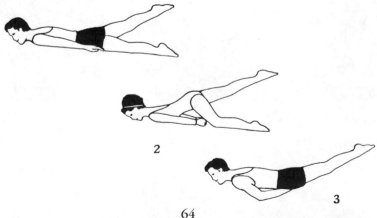

2

3

Modified Push-ups

BENEFITS: Tones and strengthens arms and shoulders, firms bosom, increases strength and flexibility in wrists. Many women do not do the activities that promote strong arms. This is a special concern for the disabled woman who should exploit all residual capacities to be as strong as she can be. If her arms are unaffected by the disease, they may be her best asset. A man can use this pose for "definition" to help his appearance, function, and posture. Because of hormone differences, women do not get the bulky contours that men do.

TECHNIQUE: Begin from a prone position, face down, hands beneath shoulders. Separate the knees slightly; bend the knees so that the lower leg forms a 45 degree angle with the thigh. Hold the back straight so that it doesn't bend at the waist. Inhale, and press evenly against the floor as you straighten the arms. Exhale as you lower the body slowly to the starting position. Repeat until you are tired. Take equal time to recoup. Increase repetitions as your strength increases.

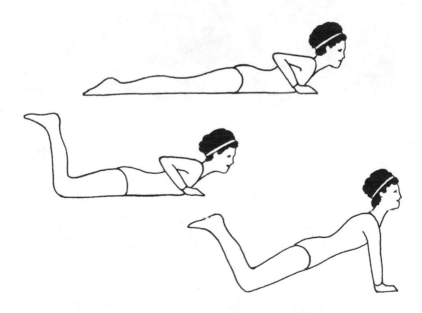

The Swan

BENEFITS: This pose warms the spinal column, preparing it for more vigorous backbending poses such as Cobra. Because the arms control the amount of strength, this is the ideal way for the beginner to experience the exhilarating effects of spinal flexibility. A counterpose is built into this movement, so it doesn't require another position to bring the body back into balance.

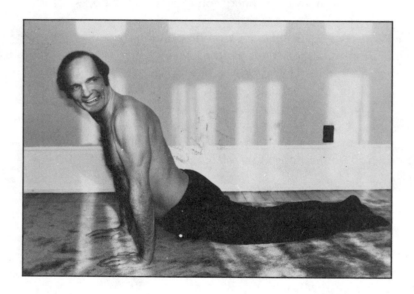

TECHNIQUE: From a prone position, push up to hands-and knees with the shoulders directly over the hands, hips over knees. To gently play with your spine's capacity for stretch, drop your hips and pelvis toward the mat. Here you are creating a concave arc in your spine; then press up through hands-and-knees, to child pose, rounding the back in a convex line. Alternately dip and fold the pelvis, watching the breath, and allowing it to flow freely as you move.

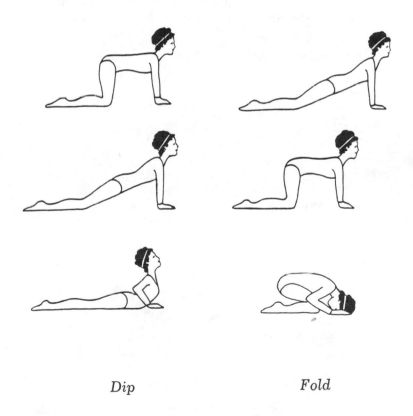

Dip   *Fold*

Bow

BENEFITS: Bow does all the stretching and toning that Cobra does with a bonus of a thigh stretch and added leverage through the arms which opens the chest and upper back. Especially recommended for the round-shouldered student.

BOW WARM-UP: From a prone position, bend one knee with your heel toward your buttocks. Reach back and grip the ankle with the hand on that side. If it is not within your grasp, a belt or sock can be wrapped around it giving you the leverage you need. Gently squeeze the buttocks together and lift the foot and knee upward as you inhale. The knee should come off the floor as high as possible. Be aware of the stretch your "quads" and low back are comfortable with. As you arch your back, lift the head and keep the arms straight. Exhale, lower the body face down, and relax. Reverse sides, noticing any differences in the two sides. Balance is a little tricky at first, so don't be disturbed if you falter.

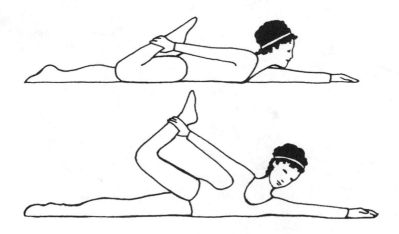

BILATERAL BOW: From the prone position, bring both heels toward the buttocks. The knees of the beginner can be separated. Knees should be closer together as you progress. Grip the ankles, inhale, and lift the feet high. The legs should actively resist the hands, pulling away, creating a truly isometric movement. This brings both elasticity and strength to the spine. In the beginning, hold the pose only for the length of the inhale/lift. As you progress, hold a little longer, breathing in the pose. Release slowly. Relax completely. Enjoy.

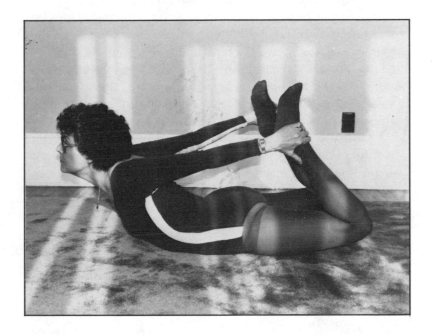

The Bridge

BENEFITS: This pose stretches and strengthens the knees and the thigh muscles. The back is given a controlled arch, which tones the muscles in the lumbo-sacral area. It also stretches the muscles of the abdomen, a very pleasant sensation, if these muscles are tight from working on abdominal toning, or if the student has abdominal cramping. As spinal flexibility increases, the chest opens and the stretch is felt in the ribs.

TECHNIQUE: From a resting position on your back, bring the shoulders together and down, moving the shoulder blades toward one another. Bend the knees, and position the feet on the floor beneath the knees. The feet should be at least the width of the hips apart. Exhale from this position, and as the inhale occurs, press the buttocks together and upward, lifting the tailbone and each vertebra of the spinal column in a rolling sequential manner. Arms can lie palms down beside the hips, or, to increase leverage and lift the arch higher, the hands can grip the ankles. Do the first effort gently, and hold only until the breath dictates an exhale. The next effort can be more vigorous, and held for several breaths, to build stamina and magnify the asana's effects. As always, rest well after the pose, focusing upon the changes you observe in the body.

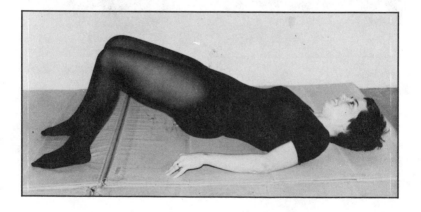

T-Twist

BENEFITS: This is a very popular pose because the after effects are so pleasant. The muscles of the waist, hips, and shoulders get a very stimulating stretch. The spinal column is flexed in a torque-like manner, increasing mobility, as well as creating space between the vertebrae. The organs of excretion, the kidneys, bowel, pancreas, and gall bladder, benefit from the increased supply of blood. Even the neck gets a revitalizing massage, releasing tension dynamically.

TECHNIQUE: Lie on your back with arms extended straight out from the shoulders in a "T" position. Turn the head and look at your right hand, palm down, on the floor. Bring the right foot up to knee level, and then over the extended left leg, placing it outside the left knee. Keep the shoulders flat as you place the left hand on the outside of the right knee and roll the right knee toward the floor. (Face and palm are opposite directions of the knee and lever arm). The breath will be restricted, so effort must be made to breathe as you hold . . . at least 15 seconds, before slowly releasing, observing, and reversing.

NOTE: Although this pose is great anytime the back is tight or "complaining," it is especially nice in bed to ease morning stiffness. Also helpful is a sensitive friend, who can provide gentle leverage by holding shoulder and opposite knee to the floor or bed, adding to the stretch.

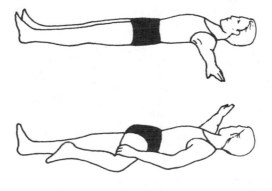

71

Knees-To-Side Twist

BENEFITS: Same as for T-twist, in a gentler, easier-to-remember form. Tones the abdominal muscles.

TECHNIQUE: On the back in a T position, extend the arms, palms down, straight out from the shoulders. Bend the knees and bring the feet close to the buttocks. Inhale with the body centered. Exhale, as you roll knees and face simultaneously in opposite directions. Hold. Inhale and return to center; then exhale with the stretch in the opposite direction. Do several cycles, taking care that the shoulders remain flat, and the breath dictates movement.

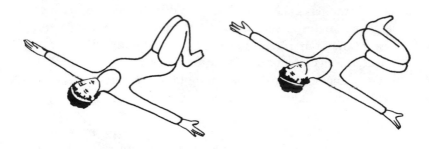

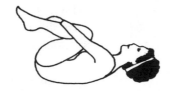

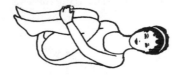

Knee Hug

BENEFITS: The knee hug is a restorative pose. It stretches the low back muscles across the rounded surface of the back, ironing them out beneath the weight of the body. Further pressure is added by clasping the arms across the folded knees. It is also good for relieving the bloated feeling after foods which don't quite agree with one.

TECHNIQUE: Lying on your back, flex the knees to the chest, encircle them with clasped arms, and squeeze gently. If the abdomen is bulky, part the knees. A gentle rolling back and forth or side to side may feel good. Stretch, squeeze, enjoy.

Ceiling Walk

BENEFITS: Because the back is flat, the strain of postural alignment is eliminated, making the ceiling walk safe for even the student with a weak, problem back. This is basically an abdominal strengthener, but the muscles which flex the hip joints and raise the thighs are also toned. Abdominal muscles do more than hold the stomach in. Functions include balancing the opposing muscles in the back which hold the spine straight, moving the bowels, urinating, childbirth, even exhalation requires contraction of these diverse muscle groups.

TECHNIQUE: Lie flat on a mat as you raise both legs perpendicular to the floor. Check your back at the waistline. It should be flat and pressed into the floor. With feet flat and knees straight, simulate a wide stride across the ceiling. Watch the breath and coordinate it with the alternate movements. Work until you feel a quivering sensation or grow tired. Then rest, with knees bent.

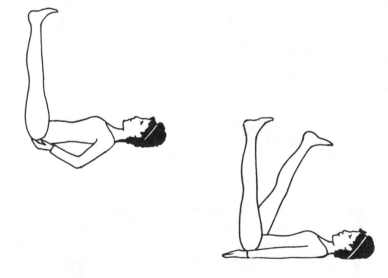

Leg Stretch

BENEFITS: This stretch provides a gentle way to keep the leg muscles supple without strenuous movements. The muscle tissue acts like a second heart, promoting circulation, and reducing the possibility of injury. It also relieves tension and stiffness, and clears the muscles of waste residues like lactic acid. Because you are on your back, improper stretching of the back is eliminated.

TECHNIQUE: Lie on your back with both legs straight. Raise one leg. Experiment with your degree of flexibility. Use a tie, sock, or rope if you cannot grip the ankle with both hands, knee straight. Remember, it isn't how far you stretch, but more the relaxed ease and awareness with which you stretch. Keep the leg on the floor straight also. Hold for at least three good breaths, then release, observe, and reverse.

NOTE: This provides you with an opportunity to focus upon a comparison of the legs. Most of us have a stronger, more flexible, favorite side. Be aware of it. Once you know which side is weaker, try to balance your bodywork so the weaker side gets more attention. ALWAYS BEGIN WITH THIS SIDE. This way, you are not exercising the weaker side based on the stronger side's limits. (This can lead to injuries.)

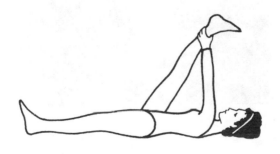

Shoulderstand

BENEFITS: It is often said "If you can find time for only one yoga pose, do the shoulderstand." Before you decide that this posture is not for you, consider Arlene, our wheelchair student. It is her favorite pose. With the help of a friend, Arlene is assisted into shoulderstand every week. (If we forget about it, she reminds us!) It counteracts the stasis of blood which occurs when one is sitting in a wheelchair, or any chair, for long periods of time.

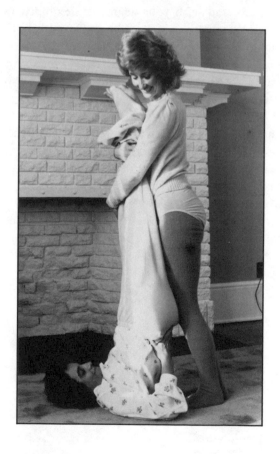

Since the body is in an inverted position, the blood flows more freely to the upper parts of the body, benefiting, especially, the brain and sense organs in the head. The heart is positioned directly above the thyroid gland, which is responsible for metabolism. This asana stimulates it directly, as well as the other glands of the endocrine system. The trunk is strengthened and the neck is stretched. This is particularly good for those who reflect their stress in muscular tension in the neck and shoulders. This asana is best known for its restorative, fatigue-relieving properties. Once the student gains strength and proficiency to hold the pose for longer periods of time, it teaches calmness of mind and body.

THIS POSE IS NOT TO BE PRACTICED BY PERSONS WITH GLAUCOMA, OR UNCONTROLLED HIGH BLOOD PRESSURE. THE STUDENT SHOULD BE WARNED AGAINST TURNING THE HEAD FROM SIDE TO SIDE WHILE IN THE POSTURE.

TECHNIQUE: Lie on your back, palms down. Slowly raise the legs, bend the knees, and roll the hips over the shoulders. Bend the elbows and support the back with the hands at the waist. Then bring the hands lower on the trunk (toward the floor) as you extend the legs upward. Try to stretch the legs high and straighten the back. Position the heels over an imaginary plumb line which would go through the pelvis to the shoulders. Hold, then release slowly as you roll back down to the floor with control. Allow the body to relax completely.

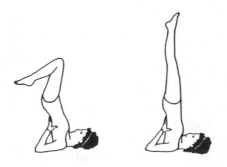

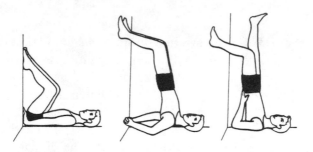

MODIFICATIONS: If strength, body weight, or balance limit the accomplishment of shoulderstand, use a wall or table as a help. Position the hips very close to a wall/floor junction. Stretch the legs upward, bend the knees, and adjust the angle of the body with pressure from the feet. Lift one leg from the wall ceilingward, if it feels right. Then reverse the legs, being patient and cautious. Align the legs with the wall, observe the circulatory changes, and roll gently down. An assistant may be necessary to steady this pose, but it should not be omitted due to pride. There's too much to gain.

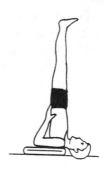

NOTE: Frequently a student with rigid, tight neck and shoulders will experience pain in the neck during and after this pose. This is because the weight is being improperly borne on the neck. (It's called a shoulderstand, not a neck stand!) This can usually be remedied by placing a firm folded blanket under the shoulders and back. The neck should be free and without weight or pressure. The elbows or arms can be pressed closer to each other, giving the shoulders a higher base of support.

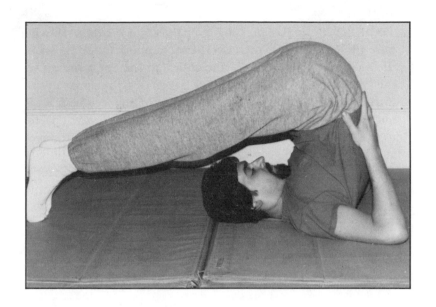

Plough

BENEFITS: This position stretches the posterior surface of the body from the heels through the back of the neck. The effects of gravity are reversed, and the abdomen is drawn in, massaging and rejuvenating the organs within. The angle of flexion at the neck promotes extra circulation from the carotid and jugulars, as well as the regular supply from the vertebral arteries, flooding the areas of the thyroid, parathyroid, pituitary, and pineal glands. The organs of sense in the head, as well as the brain itself, receive an increase in blood flow which rejuvenates and improves their function. This is a balanced stretch, which has the outward appearance of stillness, but it tones your awareness as you watch yourself adjust the balance throughout the body and observe the effects. The breath is full and steady, calming the mind to relaxation and observation.

This asana is specifically therapeutic for back problems, constipation, tightness of the neck and hamstrings, glandular imbalances, abdominal fat, and "hangover" headaches.

TECHNIQUE: Lie flat, pressing the palms into the floor. Slowly raise the legs straight, then overhead. Support the spine with the hands at the waist. Press the chin into the chest and bring the shoulder blades close together, protecting the upper neck. If the feet don't touch the floor, a stool or pillow can be placed under them. Keep the knees straight. (Students who are unable to extend their legs can enjoy this pose with the knees dropped at either side of the ears). Hold this pose as long as you like: Twenty seconds to five minutes. Then, supporting your hips with your hands, press upper through lower vertebrae into the floor as you unfold with control. Keep the head on the floor and the legs straight and together. Rest and observe. ALWAYS FOLLOW THIS POSE WITH "FISH."

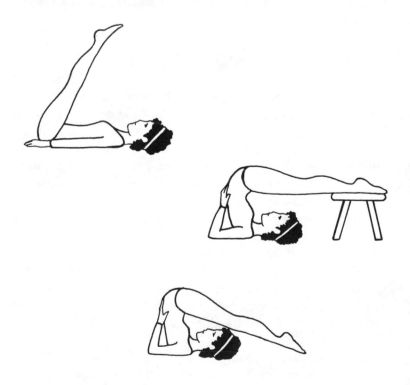

Fish

BENEFITS: This posture is called Fish because of the way it opens the chest, superinflating the lungs, thus making the body more buoyant. This pose is considered a "counterpose" to shoulderstand and plough. It counteracts stiffness of the neck and compensates for bending the head severely forward. It is a valuable tool for respiratory training. It is therapeutic for the shallow breather, the student with emphysema or asthma. The chest is thrown open, accentuating deep abdominal breathing. A gentle arch of the back gives the spine an easy stretch, making it especially adaptable to the stiff beginner. Because of the way it stretches the stomach, it is sometimes effective in curbing nausea.

TECHNIQUE: From a relaxed position on your back, place your hands under your buttocks, palms up. As you press your elbows into the floor, open and lift your sternum, or breastbone. Lift the chin and arch the neck backward, resting the top of the head on the mat. Weightbearing should be easily felt on the crown of the head, the elbows, the hands and hips, and along the extended legs. The shoulders and face should be free and passive, and emphasis should be on filling the great space created in the chest with a fresh current of breath. Come out of the pose by easing the chest higher, taking weight off the head, and bringing the head, neck and shoulders to rest on the mat.

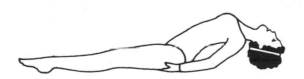

Tree (On Back)

BENEFITS: Students with vision impairment, or with decreased sensation in the feet, have difficulty with balance. These students, as well as those who are unable to stand, can practice TREE on their backs. At first, this may appear to be a compromise, but all levels of students should practice this variation occasionally. The floor will teach you to focus attention on a well-aligned spinal column, and to open at the pelvis/hip joint. This pose also extends the shoulder joints, as the palms meet in prayer position overhead, opening and expanding the ribcage, and allowing the student to experience full, deep, abdominal and complete breathing.

TECHNIQUE: Align the body, being especially aware of the surface of the mat against the back. Draw one leg up to a high stretch, so that the sole of the foot rests against the inner thigh parallel to the floor. Press the pelvis flat, and allow gravity to open the hip joint, as the knee relaxes toward the floor. Rest and observe the stretch which you can experience more fully without fear of falling. Lift the arms to an overhead prayer position, thumbs touching the mat. Breathe deeply, abdominally. Reverse sides.

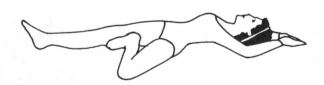

Modified Sit-Ups

BENEFITS: Weakness of the abdominal muscles is an almost universal symptom of the M.S. student. However, improving abdominal muscle tone is vital for all Gentle Yoga students. Regular sit-ups are usually too difficult, but these three variations should be easier and more workable depending on your unique abilities. Do what you can with a regular commitment.

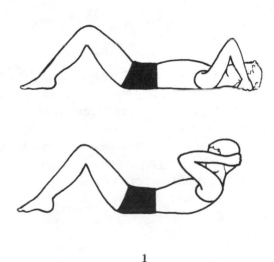

1

TECHNIQUE: #1 (The CURL) Lie on your back with legs bent, feet tucked under a couch if you like. The angle at the knee should be about 45 degrees. Clasp the hands behind the head, and as you exhale, slowly curl head and shoulders off the floor. Hold. Then inhale slowly as you roll back down. Work until you are tired, and then rest well! (If this doesn't present a challenge to you, add a small weight, maybe a book or small can of food to each hand.)

#2 (The CRUNCH) Lie on your back with feet resting on the seat of a chair, thighs perpendicular to the floor. With hands clasped behind head, roll up trying to touch your knees with your elbows. Don't be dismayed if they don't touch! The direction is what counts, not the distance. By using both straight movements and diagonal movements (elbow to opposite knee), several muscle groups are toned in the same pose. Don't forget, inhale while flat, exhale up. This way the diaphragm and "abs" are working together.

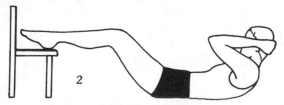

#3 The beginning position of this pose looks like the letter X: Lie on your back, arms and legs extended wide. Inhale. Raise alternate arm and leg to meet over the middle of your body as you exhale. Inhale and lie back down. Then try the other side. The supporting arm can be helping the trunk to sit up if needed. This variation is very dynamic, so approach it with attention to your limits. As you practice, observe how the limits of your strength and stretch change. This ever-changing self will keep your yoga fresh.

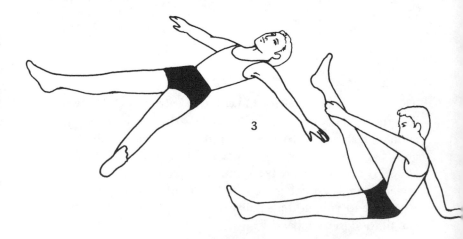

Stick Pose (Using A Wall)

BENEFITS: This pose teaches the student the correct alignment for forward bending. Forward bends are necessary to treat tightness in the backs of the legs, (the "hamstrings"). Most beginning students have this problem. Also, it is important that the student understands, both mentally and physically, how to protect the back by keeping it straight, and stick pose serves this purpose. Lastly, by elevating the legs above the level of the heart, the veins in the legs are drained and extra circulation is sent to the brain, face and endocrine system. This also teaches patience!

TECHNIQUE: Place the buttocks and soles of the feet in fetal position against a wall. Then roll from the side to the back, extend the legs up the wall, with the hands supporting the knees if needed. Relax! Enjoy this pleasant stretch, deep breathe, and visualize all the benefits of the pose. If the inner thigh muscles are also tight part the legs gently, and notice how gravity augments this stretch.

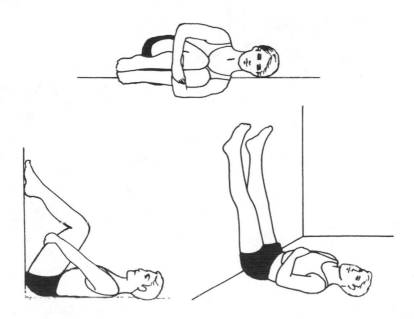

From A Wheelchair

All of the following poses should be practiced by everyone studying yoga, but we find these especially well adapted to the student confined to a wheelchair. They are also suitable for the "senior" student, as well as the sedentary office worker.

If you are doing the movements from a wheelchair, apply your brakes. If possible, sit forward so you can rest your feet on the floor, not the chair's foot support. Always remember that the chair is used for safety and mobility, not back support. Unless you have upper body involvement, make a conscious effort to sit regally straight, away from the back of the chair as much as you are able.

Much valuable bodywork can be done from a wheelchair. However, if an assistant is available, if at all possible, augment your practice with bodywork on the mat.

> *Resolve to move everything you are able to move with regular persistence. As Hippocrates said: "That which is used develops and that which is not used wastes away."*

Neck Rolls

BENEFITS: Provides range of motion lubrication to the joints of the neck. Tension in the neck and shoulders can be relieved as the neck becomes more resilient, and you experience the joy of a relaxed neck. This also firms the chin and throat.

TECHNIQUE: Sit comfortably straight, as you inhale in the upright position. Then, as you exhale slowly, allow your head to drop forward and bring your chin toward your chest. Without straining, feel the muscles along the back of the neck stretch. Inhale as you bring the head up, and exhale it to a side stretch; ear-toward-shoulder. Inhale it up, and drop your head backward gently as you raise your chin. (Support the head with your hands if needed.) These four movements test the elasticity of your neck and may be very different from one day to the next.

If you had no pain in any of these movements begin a deep breath as you roll the head around in a circular clockwise, then counter-clock-wise direction. It is helpful if a full rotation is coordinated with one complete inhale/exhale breath. At first it is common to hear popping and gritty noises which subside after faithful practice. This has such pleasant after-effects, many students practice neck rolls at odd moments throughout their day.

Leg Lifts

BENEFITS: Tones the thighs, stretches the hamstrings, tones and strengthens the hips and abdominals, relieves tired back muscles.

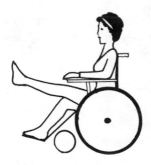

TECHNIQUE: Hold onto your chair by the sides or the seat, and extend one leg straight out and as high up as you are able. Hold for a moment, and slowly lower it. Repeat on the other side, and rest. If it seems right, .lift both legs together, then slowly lower to the floor, as you exhale. Repeat as often as needed to produce the feeling of having worked the muscles well.

The Spinal Twist

BENEFITS: A "torquing" rotation of the spine imparts a pleasant stretch and massage to the spinal column, abdomen, hips, and internal organs. Circulation is enhanced, especially around the organs of excretion: the kidneys and bowel. The twist provides the inactive student with a convenient method of invigorating his body from the chair. It is also an aid in slimming the hips and waistline.

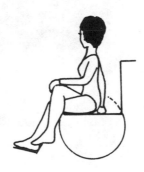

TECHNIQUE: Sit erect on the "sitting bones," and forward of the back support. Cross the legs, so the left knee is on top. Place your right hand behind you and gently twist to the left, using the right hand for leverage. Hold, rotating the upper body as far as it will comfortably go. Turn your chin over your left shoulder and look behind you. Breathe softly and hold for five breaths. Then return to center, relax, and repeat the pose in the opposite direction.

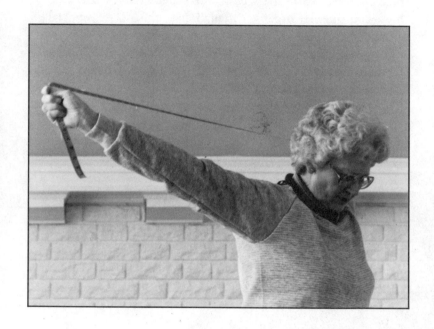

Shoulder Stretch and Shrug

BENEFITS: These movements improve the flexibility of the shoulders, upper back, and arms. It is ideal to be both flexible *and* strong. Wheelchair students use their arms a lot, and often complain of tight-jointed, stiff shoulders. These stretches are the remedy.

TECHNIQUE: Hold a necktie, rope or belt in front of you at arm's length. Keeping the arms straight, elbows locked, bring the tie over your head and behind you, widening the distance between your hands as needed. Then return hands to front. Repeat several times.

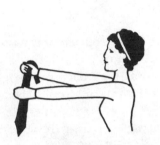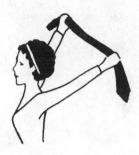

Bring both shoulders tightly up toward the shoulders. Squeeze the neck, hold, and accentuate the "uptight" posture of tension. Then release quickly, letting the shoulders drop. Feel the rush of blood to these muscles. Repeat several times.

Bend the elbows and place the hands on top of the shoulders as you rotate the elbows around in a circle. Do five circles in one direction; then reverse.

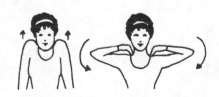

Warrior Pose

BENEFITS: This movement is a modification of a shoulder/arm stretch. Students who are round-shouldered, are developing a dowager's hump, or are stiff or muscle-bound will find this exercise helpful. This is also a useful tool in pointing out right/left imbalances.

TECHNIQUE: Use your right hand to massage and warm up the left shoulder joint. Then stretch the arm high, flexing at the elbow and palm facing the back. Bring the right arm down and up, grasping the fingers in a lock. If you can't reach, dangle a sock or scarf down from the upper hand for leverage. Remain erect as you inhale and stretch. Release, rest, reverse, and compare. Stretch more often on the tighter side.

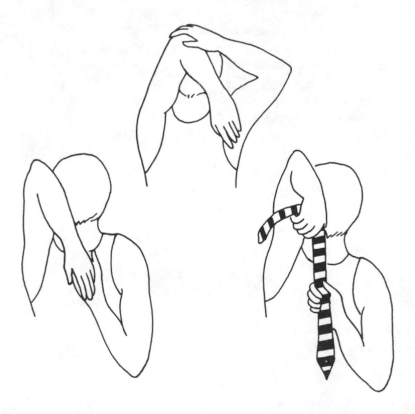

The Hand Warmer

BENEFITS: This is an excellent breathing movement, which opens the chest to the greatest amount of life-giving oxygen. It awakens the body with a tingling renewal of circulation, and is especially recommended for cold, stiff hands.

TECHNIQUE: Sitting straight, slowly inhale, and stretch the arms upward. Complete the inhalation, hold, and position the hands with palms up, toward the ceiling, *with a tight 90 degree angle at the wrists.* Be sure the arms remain straight at the elbow. As you exhale, slowly lower the arms, while maintaining the tight wrist angle. Let the arms hang passive and limp. Enjoy the after effects. Repeat.

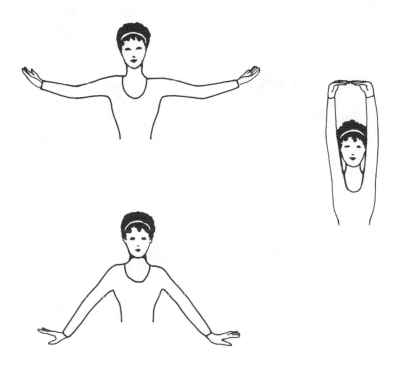

Hands

BENEFITS: Every part of your body needs exercise: stretching, increased circulation, range of motion joint treatment, strengthening. The joints farthest from the heart are first to show signs of aging. Activity counteracts this. Following are a variety of hand movements.

Massage, stretch, and move each joint in all directions.

Shake them out! Relax the wrist joint, and loosely shake floppy hands till they feel like rubber.

Make tight fists and wide open stretches.

The palm press puts pressure on the wrists and chest wall.

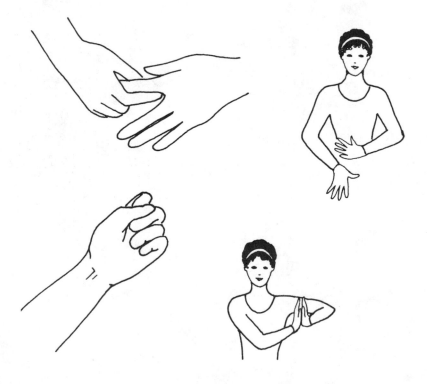

Finger Lift

BENEFITS: Strengthens the muscles on the top surface of the hand, and stretches the muscles and tendons of the palm. This will keep the joints healthier by balancing the muscles which move them more evenly, preventing clawlike deformity.

TECHNIQUE: Rest your palm on a flat surface. Then stiffen and contract the fingers up, away from that surface, as high as you are able. Hold for the count of ten, then relax and repeat . . . do both hands.

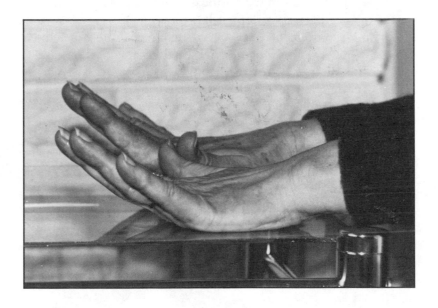

The Perineal Exercise

BENEFITS: Increases muscle tone and circulation to the reproductive system and the pelvic floor. Miriam Ottenberg, in her book *In Pursuit Of Hope,* believes this is a vital tool in controlling urinary problems in the MSer. It is an aid when poor muscle tone is the cause of hemorrhoids, constipation, prostrate enlargement, and prolapsed uterus. It also should be practiced during pregnancy and after childbirth to tone supportive muscles.

TECHNIQUE: Sit comfortably; inhale. As you exhale slowly, contract the muscles of the buttocks, squeezing and tightening as if to hold back urination. Hold, then inhale and relax. At first, these movements may be subtle. If you can't feel the muscles responding, squeeze the seat muscles together, and watch for the pelvis to rise slightly as the buttocks muscles firm. Another way to practice is to start and stop the flow of urine, repeatedly, midstream, in your bladder elimination. Proficiency gradually increases with practice. Remember, contract and hold on the exhalation; relax and rest on the inhalation.

This is one exercise which can be practiced unobtrusively, anywhere. Students can practice this by utilizing time ordinarily spent waiting. Many students like to practice this while sitting in the bathtub.

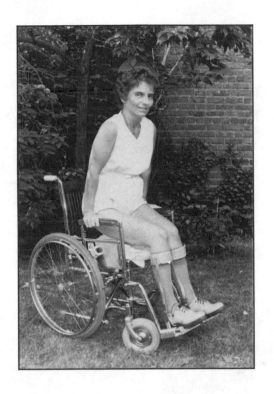

Wheelchair Pushup

BENEFITS: This maintains the arm and shoulder strength so necessary in transfering the wheelchair student from chair to car, stool, or bed. Rather than wait until these movements are critical to getting around, why not warm them up and strengthen them several times during the day? This also allows air to circulate around pressure sores.

TECHNIQUE: With hands back on the arm rest even with the hips, push down extending the elbow to an almost straight position and hold for several seconds. Lower the hips slowly, with as much control as possible. Repeat until tired.

Foot Flap

BENEFITS: This movement tones the shin muscles, the ones responsible for lifting the dragging toe of foot drop. It also stretches out tight or cramping calf muscles.

TECHNIQUE: Lift and "flap" each toe, bringing it as high toward the face as possible. Release, and continue until tired.

NOTE: Most M.S. and stroke students have a weaker side. This usually will be the side which drags, especially when tired. If the student cultivates this movement with regularity, strength and function will be maximized.

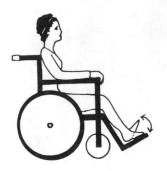

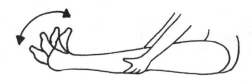

Eye Exercises

BENEFITS: Everyone can benefit from eye exercises. However, they are especially important for M.S. people because of their special eye problems. The eyes are part of the nervous system, and previously were thought to be out of our control. However, many optometrists are now using yoga techniques, illustrating that sight is capable of changing. Problems due to muscular weakness are especially benefitted by exercises which emphasize focusing, moving the eyes together as a team, and eye movement skills.

Stress affects vision through eye muscles, causing imbalances. It pulls the eyeball unevenly, just as it causes tension in the neck or jaw. An awareness of this, the use of visualization to increase circulation, and breathing techniques for stress reduction make up the natural holistic approach of treatment to improve eyesight.

General actions helpful to vision are:

* Avoid staring. Staring produces stress and immobility.

* Avoid overstimulating, i.e. too much TV.

* Hold your head parallel to the horizon. Tilting your head provokes oblique astigmatism.

* Bask your eyes in warm sunlight with lids closed.

* Massage the boney orbit of your eyes. Massage the base of the neck near the skull. Practice "palming."

* Eat carrots, sweet potatoes and leafy green vegetables, all high in vitamin A.

* Practice blinking regularly. This negates staring and washes the eyeball with tears.

* Open the eyes wide when doing the exercises. This helps to relieve tension and pressure on the eyeball.

* Relax and regulate the breath during the exercises.

EYE MOVEMENTS:

1. Sit erect, regulate the breath, and move only the eyes. Stretch them as far as possible to the right, hold for a moment, then stretch as far as possible to the left, holding. A definite stretch should be felt. Repeat several times. Beginners should increase work gradually.

2. Next, stretch eyes upward as far as they will move, hold; then downward, and hold. (You should be able to see parts of the hair, nose, and lap.)

3. Move eyes from a maximum stretch to the upper right on a diagonal line to the lower left. Check that you're not holding your breath. Repeat several times. Then move from lower right point to the upper left. Use rhythmic control, as opposed to quick jerks. Repeat movements so that all four points are used at least twice.

4. Slowly circle the eyes clockwise, rolling them around the edges of your field of vision. Focus on objects and use them to pull the eyes to a maximum stretch. THE MOVEMENTS MUST BE SMOOTH AND SLOW. As you increase proficiency, circle more rapidly, but don't allow jerking or dot-to-dot movements. Rest when tired, lids closed, observing the effects of your work. Then roll your eyes counterclockwise.

5. To practice changing focus, hold your arm out straight with thumb pointed upward. Position thumb-nail in front of an object in the distance—at least 20 feet away. Then rapidly move your focus from your thumb to the object: thumb; object; etc. Follow with palming: create intense friction and heat between your hands by briskly rubbing palms together. Place the warm palms over the closed eyes, completely obliterating light. Bathe them in the warm velvet blackness.

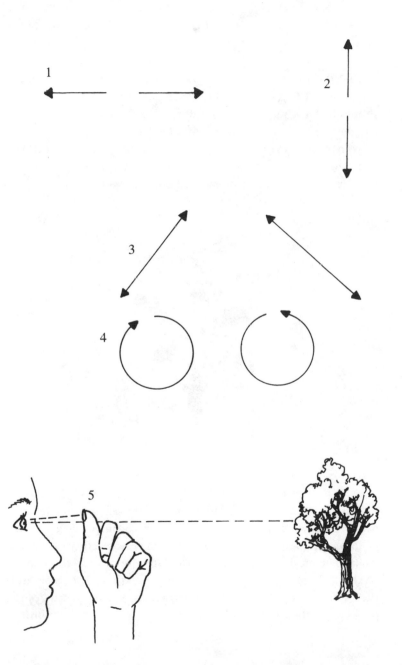

Candle Gazing

BENEFITS: As well as clarifying the vision and washing away impurities, this exercise trains the mind in concentration.

TECHNIQUE: Sit a few feet away from a candle at eye level. Stare into the flame with as little blinking as possible. Your gaze should be steady for about 3 minutes. As the eyes begin to water, gently close them, "palm," and hold the image of the flame in your mind's eye. The image will be retained on the retina. Hold the image as long as you can, bringing it back to center as it fades. This exercise stimulates the nerve centers.

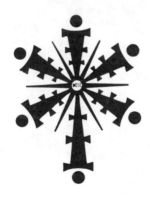

The use of a Mandala or circular chart designed to stimulate and exercise muscles and nerves for corrective purposes is an ancient technique. The chart above is a miniature copy of such a chart. The student is instructed to place the nose in the center of the full sized chart and move the eyes first clockwise and then counterclockwise around the outer edges of the design. As proficiency develops, move inward a tier along each arm of the figure.

Abdominal Lift

BENEFITS: The Sanskrit name for this asana is Udyana Bhanda, literally "flying up and binding"—which describes the action of the diaphragm. The breath is exhaled from the body, the airway closed, and a vacuum created in the respiratory space. This vacuum pulls the abdominal muscles internally, massaging the organs within the trunk. The most obvious benefits of this pose are noticed by students with constipation. A vigorous massage from this asana every morning stimulates a sluggish colon to renew regularity. The muscles of the abdomen and diaphragm grow stronger and become more efficient at breathing, movement, and supporting the anterior surface of the body. Many students notice a trimmer waistline after practicing this pose for a few months. There is a profound effect on circulation as blood is compressed and then released from the large major blood vessels which go through the interior midline of the body. This is accompanied by a pleasant sensation of freshly oxygenated blood flooding through the trunk, sparking your total being with an "energy cocktail."

TECHNIQUE: Beginners assume a spread-leg stance, hands on thighs, with arms supporting some of the weight of the body. (As the student practices, the effort becomes second nature, and seated, kneeling, even hands-and-knees positions serve just as well.) With an audible "haaaaa" sound, exhale all the air you can from your lungs. Quickly close the lips and don't allow air to refill the lungs. With this maneuver, a vacuum is created in the torso. Before you need a breath, LIFT UPWARD AND INWARD with the belly. With practice, you will see that you can create a great hollow within the rib cage. A noticeable suction is also apparent at the base of the throat. When you need to breathe, release the lift. An inhale breath occurs spontaneously. Rest and take a moment to study the after-effects upon the body. When the "rush" has subsided, repeat twice. After you feel confident in the one lift, try expelling three successive breaths with no inhalation, with a lift after each one. These additional lifts expel the residual air from the lungs, which rarely is exchanged. This also magnifies the effects of the pose.

V

Stress Management: Relaxation and Visualization

Stress is a common problem which affects all of us. It is caused by constant changes in a constantly changing world, and there's no escape. Even our language recognizes the problem: the word *uptight* is now included in Webster's Dictionary—and we all know exactly what it means without reading the definition.

Stress is constant and cumulative, and it doesn't take something traumatic like a tornado or a death in the family to cause it. It can be caused by starting a new job as well as losing a job, by marriage or divorce, by acquiring a new family member or by a child leaving home, by starting or stopping school, by buying a home or selling one, by sickness, retirement, vacation, or even by Christmas! When you add the run-of-the-mill stressors such as noise, air pollution, alcohol, tobacco, drugs, poor diet, hatred, anxiety, fear, frustration, a crabby boss, a crying baby, a rebellious teenager, or a demanding parent, you begin to realize that we are actually bombarded by stress. From the time we jump out of bed when the alarm clock jangles, to the time we turn off the late-night news, stress is pummeling and pounding us from all directions.

Our response to stress has three stages. First comes the stage when blood pressure rises, blood sugar surges, stomach acid increases, and arteries tighten. The body prepares to fight or take flight. In the second stage, the pituitary and adrenaline glands respond by pouring forth hormones. In the third stage, the body is left exhausted and spent.

We all experience these phases, and we know instinctively that our bodies suffer from the process. Doctors tell us that unrelieved stress will eventually cause a body breakdown, usually in the body's weakest area.

We know that high blood pressure, heart attacks, strokes, ulcers, migraine headaches, and colitis are the results of stress. Stress can antagonize M.S.; people often suffer set-backs during or after periods of stress in their lives. And new studies point to stress as a possible cause of arthritis. In fact, the American Medical Association now reports that 80% of *all* diseases are related in some way to stress.

Yoga, of course, cannot eliminate stress from our lives, but it can overcome tension and mental strain and restore order to the body-mind. For thousands of years, yoga has emphasized relaxation; many people first discover yoga in their search for knowledge about relaxation.

In four very basic ways, yoga offers relief from stress:

1. Yoga teaches the care and appreciation of the body which in turn discourages bad habits. This eliminates some of the most basic stressors in our lives.

2. Yoga emphasizes a serene life style. It changes values and simplifies life. It directs the mind away from

harmful stress, looks at life positively, and creates a calm core.

3. Yoga's physical postures emphasize slow stretching. Stretching releases tension in tight muscles and joints.

4. Yoga teaches its age-old relaxation and deep breathing techniques.

People with disabilities appreciate the ability to relax. As a M.S. yoga student said, "I had no idea how to relax before I took yoga. In fact, I doubt if I'd ever been really relaxed in my life. Now whenever I feel myself getting tense, I tell my muscles to relax."

Another Gentle Yoga student's experience: "My grandmother and I were very close. When she died, I was so afraid I'd have an exacerbation. But whenever I felt myself getting tense, especially at the funeral, I did my deep breathing and told myself to relax and I got along without any problems at all."

Each yoga session ends with deep relaxation. The student reclines on his back with eyes closed, feet slightly apart, hands at sides with palms turned upward. The consciousness is directed slowly and deliberately to every area of the body. The student becomes aware of each area, feeling it acutely and relaxing it, searching carefully for any tension or tightness. This is a slow deliberate process of observing and "letting go." The body becomes totally relaxed and tension free. The benefits are unbelievable to anyone who has not experienced this. It is a firm yoga rule: Relaxation is NEVER omitted at the end of a yoga session.

A relaxation script follows. We suggest that you either ask someone to read it for you, or tape your own voice. It should be read softly and very slowly.

Script for Relaxation

This is your time. There is nowhere you need to go and nothing you need to do. These next minutes will be devoted to your health and well-being. Be aware that the day's events and problems will wait as you settle into a comfortable position of rest, and retreat into your inner dimension. Transfer your mind from all other spaces to the space your body is occupying. Do not allow the frenzied feelings of your day to intrude as you retreat into stillness.

Breathe deeply as you would in a heavy sleep. With each breath, direct your thoughts to your muscles. Nothing else matters. Allow nothing to disturb you.

Make a rigid hard fist with your right hand. Then press the forearm downward toward the floor. Press the arm toward the body, squeezing tightly. Hold. Now release with a sigh. Take a moment to observe that arm and hand. Compare. Now shift your attention to your left hand. Make a fist. Now press the forearm toward the floor, pressing in toward the body, squeezing tightly— Harder. Release with a sigh.

Purse your lips into an O. Now spread your lips as you open your mouth widely. Yawn and let your jaw hang slack. Take a deep breath and let it go. Raise your forehead as though in surprise. Harder. Now furrow your brow as though worried. Release with a deep exhalation. Observe how warm and heavy your facial muscles feel. Enjoy the sensation. Inhale deeply and bring your shoulders up toward your ears. Tightly. Harder. Then release and exhale. Observe. Do it again. Rearrange your shoulders in a comfortable position. Feel the

heavy warm sensation of relaxation spreading through-
out your upper body. With each new breath, you feel
more relaxed, more at rest, more peaceful. Now tense
your right leg. Release. Tense your left leg. Release. Point
the toes of each foot toward the face, stretching from the
heel to the calf. Relax.

Surrender your entire body to feelings of refreshing re-
laxation. Feel each breath flood your body with tran-
quillity, washing away all tension. Saturate your lungs
with sparkling beautiful energy. With each breath, expe-
rience a deeper feeling of letting go. Remember this
place of peace and strength within you.

Now reacquaint yourself with your surroundings.
Open your eyes, stretch, smile, sit up slowly.

Keep this pleasant feeling with you throughout your
day. Use this feeling as the basis for comparison when
you begin to feel tense.

Visualization

The use of visualization as a tool for body-mind man-
agement and healing has been receiving a great deal of attention lately. Such people as Norman Cousins, Dr.
Herbert Benson, Dr. Carl Simonton, and Marcus Bach—as
well as the Menninger Clinic and the entire fields of bio-
feedback, autogenic therapy, and holistic health—have
focused new attention on the ability of the mind to aid in
the healing process.

In yoga, relaxation and visualization have been used for
centuries to promote healing and well-being. In fact, in
modern scientific studies, yogis have been carefully ex-

amined and studied because of their ability to control their heart rates and body temperatures.

In his work with cancer patients, Dr. Carl Simonton is attracting world-wide attention by demonstrating that by visualization a person can play a role in curing disease. He begins by teaching the patient to relax with techniques similar to those used in yoga. The patient is then given a complete explanation of his immune mechanism and of the treatments he will be receiving. At the end of each training session, the patient relaxes and visualizes himself in a well state. Patients who follow the plan diligently and are enthusiastic about it, show marked improvement.

In bio-feedback clinics all across America, patients are being taught to control their blood pressure and headaches. Studies in Pennsylvania have shown that patients can raise the number of immune cells in their blood by as much as 18%. And in Colorado, bone healing after ski fractures is greatly accelerated through visualization techniques.

There is every reason for students of Gentle Yoga to practice and benefit from using visualization techniques. As visualization is practiced, it becomes possible for the student to actually think warmth and energy into any specific area of the body. Of course, practice makes perfect— and it takes practice to perfect this ability, but we must NEVER UNDERESTIMATE the ability of our own body-minds to heal and regenerate.

A script for visualization follows:

Script for Visualization

Before you begin this period of relaxation, choose one area of the body upon which you want to concentrate healing. It may be an arm, a shoulder, a knee, a leg—some area which has been a trouble spot for you. Recline on your back.

Roll your head from side to side. Let all tension leave your body. Relax your forehead and your eyes. Relax your cheeks and your nose. Relax your mouth and let your chin droop. Relax the muscles of your neck. Relax your chest, your waist, your abdomen. Let your body sink and flatten onto the floor. Relax your hips, your thighs, your knees. Let your feet feel limp and soft, as though they are unattached. Allow your whole body to feel limp and loose and free of all tension. Observe the silence of your mind and listen only to your breathing. Watch the cycles of your breath as each breath begins— and ends. Breathe in cycles. Observe how each breath begins and how it ends. Breathe deeply, letting the air fill your abdomen with warm, clean, clear, healing energy-laden oxygen.

Now, after your next inhalation, direct that inhaled energy into the area to be healed. Breathe in. As you exhale, transfer the warmth and energy to the area. Feel its warmth as it fills the area with healing, sparkling, vibrating energy. Inhale again. Feel the energy flooding the area with healing light. Inhale. Feel the warmth rush into the area, washing away tension and tightness, loosening and cleaning, healing with oxygen, light, air, energy. Continue. With each inhalation, transfer healing to the area.

Now, in your mind, see the area to be healed as healthy and perfect. Picture each detail. Mentally superimpose this picture above the physical area of yourself and see them merge. Continue breathing, deeply, quietly, holding this vision.

Now, slowly stretch. Yawn. When you are ready, open your eyes. Observe the renewed feeling of your body. Keep it with you throughout the rest of your day.

Your food
shall be your medicine
&
your medicine
shall be your
food

—Hippocrates, 424 B.C.

VI

Nutrition the Yoga Way

Our American diet of hot dogs, apple pie, pop and you-never-outgrow-your-need-for-milk has gone sour! With 50% of our elderly suffering from chronic diseases, 50% of our deaths directly attributed to damaging lifestyles, and almost half of our population overweight, we are in serious need of better nutritional habits. Heart disease, cancer of the colon and breast, stroke, high blood pressure, diabetes, arteriosclerosis and cirrhosis of the liver have all been linked to the American diet. Yet we surely have an abundance of guidance: Magical diets fill our bookstores, and every magazine, newspaper, and TV talk show offers advice. There are diets from the Air Force and from the Mayo Clinic. There's the Atkins diet, the Stillman diet, the Pritikin diet, the Scarsdale diet, a brown rice diet, a grapefruit diet, and even a water diet. The subjects of nutrition and weight maintenance become more confusing each day.

Crash diets are not the answer. Approximately 20 million Americans will embark on diets this year, but four out of five people who lose weight will regain it. These crash diets enable people to lose pounds because they remove all the options. This controls the choices, but as soon as "normal" eating habits are resumed, weight is quickly regained. Crash diets not only don't last, they can be hazardous to your health. A yo-yo pattern will continue until there is a permanent decision to alter food habits and the attitudes affecting them.

The yoga approach to nutrition is simple, natural, and based on common sense. It can be explained with these basic concepts:

1. Eat only when hungry.
2. Eat sparingly of high-nutrition foods.
3. Eat pure, fresh, raw, unprocessed foods.
4. Drink 6-8 glasses of water daily.
5. Think of eating as refueling your body cells—not as entertainment, a reward, or a tonic for boredom.

Eat Only When Hungry

The old concept of three-squares-a-day/meat-and-potatoes/remember-the-starving-children has encouraged us to become a nation of gluttons! Imagine what the starving masses would think if they could grasp our national problem of malnutrition through overconsumption. Habits of eating by the clock should not be mistaken for hunger, which few of us actually experience. Many of us eat because everyone else is eating, or because it affords us a break. A better understanding of why we eat is a necessary step in behavior modification as it relates to food habits. Making a list of foods eaten, and when, may reveal some surprising patterns.

114

A very insightful experience can be gained by a few days on a fruit and vegetable juice fast. Before embarking on a fast, a student should be in sound nutritional health and have proper information and supervision, as well as a positive attitude toward fasting. For this reason, unsupervised fasting is not recommended for *all* students, especially those with the various and complex problems this book deals with. It is, however, an excellent tool for some students who want to overcome compulsive eating. Throughout history, people have fasted to heighten athletic or religious endeavors, and to cleanse the body of its accumulated toxins. Most people who have not fasted picture an agonizing bout with constant hunger. They are amazed to learn that after a few hours of feeling empty, hunger is totally gone. A mild ketosis occurs as the body begins to burn fats. Sensations of lightness, purification, self-mastery, and a heightened sense of well-being prevail, as well as the joy of freedom from routine meal chores. Then after a possible period of caffeine or sugar withdrawal, one learns that s/he will not perish if a meal is missed. In fact, as we grow older, we need less fuel and, if our consumption doesn't decrease, we "wear" what we eat in excess. Fasting is an important tool in the understanding of conscious eating.

Eat Sparingly of High Nutrition Foods

To do this, first become aware of your portions. Fat people actually do need more food to "fill them up" because big stomachs require more food to achieve that satisfied feeling of fullness. Another bonus of fasting is that the stomach will return to a smaller size; an alternative is to eat from a small bowl which holds smaller portions for a week until the stomach shrinks.

Eating high nutrition foods will provide new and varied taste experiences. The following are *superfoods*. See if you can eat at least one each day.

whole wheat bread	carrots
sprouts	sunflower seeds
bananas	sweet potatoes
tofu	liver
nuts	wheat germ
oranges	nutritional yeast
broccoli	apples
brown rice	yogurt
oatmeal	salmon
dried peas and beans	

Rather than focusing on the negative "can't haves," this concentration on high nutrition enables you to feel proud about what you are doing right.

Eat Pure, Fresh, Raw, Unprocessed Foods

This concept is another way of saying: Eat as high on the food chain as you can. If you consider wheat, eaten by a cow, and the cow in turn being eaten by a tiger, the tiger would be filled with the waste products of the cow as well as its nutrients, and, of course, the wheat. So nutritionally speaking, the tiger would be the least pure source for man to eat, the cow next, and the wheat would be highest on the food chain. If an effort is made to replace the less pure foods in our diet with more wholesome alternatives, we gradually eliminate processed foods like white sugar and flour, fried foods, foods with chemicals, preservatives, and hormones added. This is why many yoga students choose a modified vegetarian diet; others choose to avoid red meat.

The vegetarian question is a debatable topic. The facts are in, however: vegetarians have a reduced risk of developing heart disease, diabetes, high blood pressure, back problems, and certain kinds of cancer. In addition, studies show that vegetarians are much trimmer than their meat-eating friends. One study in Boston revealed that among 116 vegetarians and their comparison group, the vegetarians weighed an average of 33 pounds less.

Food in its least processed form is best. Fresh, raw, organically grown food is superior to frozen; frozen is more nutritious than canned; canned food is so overprocessed that its food value is diminished as much as 90%. Junk food and fabricated food which pretends to be another are harmful and misleading. Examples are the colored, fruit-flavored beverages masquerading as fruit juices. Unless the consumer reads the label, s/he would assume from the picture and the name that such a product is a nutritious food product. Eating junk food is destructive in three ways: (1) It overburdens the body with waste products, (2) It creates a compulsion for more of this addictive food, and (3) It takes the place of valuable food.

This eating principle would not be complete without mentioning a very important individual method for determining pure food: allergy testing. It has long been understood that certain individuals exhibit an intolerance for what is considered pure food. Symptoms such as wheezing or a rash after a food is eaten make this apparent. However, there are less obvious signs of food allergy which aren't as well known. They are headache, gas, irritability, nasal congestion, joint stiffness, tiredness, even bladder irritation. If sensitivity to a food is suspected, that food should be avoided. If symptoms improve or disappear, that may be enough "prevention." However, a skin test for allergies of foods most often eaten may reveal unsuspected sensitivities. The cost is well worth it; you will use the information obtained for the rest of your life.

The need to eliminate drugs should be obvious. This includes caffeine (coffee, tea, chocolate and cola), nicotine, marijuana, sleeping pills, diet pills, and any other body or mind altering drug not prescribed by a physician.

Drink 6 – 8 Glasses of Water Daily

Like air, water is one of the essential components of our physical chemistry. Insufficient intake of water is detrimental to both the kidneys and cell function. Although a large percentage of your food is water, six eight-ounce glasses should be taken every day to be sure you're getting enough to meet your body's needs. It is best not to drink iced water, as recent studies reveal a correlation between excess cold drinks and increased upper respiratory infections. Ice probably decreases the protective mucous membrane, making the throat more vulnerable. Hard water, spring water, and distilled water are preferable to the processed, softened, polluted water supplies available in many of our communities. The student who keeps his body properly hydrated will be rewarded with regular elimination and moist, fresh-looking skin.

Think of Eating as Refueling Your Body Cells

Eating is not entertainment, a reward, or a tonic for boredom, loneliness, anger, or depression. Your thinking or your attitude about your diet is the most important facet of your eating behavior. These attitudes about food come from your past conditioning, as well as your current belief system. You need to examine and rethink erroneous attitudes and replace them with positive healthful ones. When you were a child, special occasions were probably celebrated by a sweet treat, cake and ice cream for a birthday, root beer floats on Saturday night, homemade pie and candy on holidays. In your subconscious mind, you probably associate these "goodies" with happiness and fun. Yet in your adult mind, you know that they are thieves, robbing you of your health. Until you change these attitudes, your diet will be one of temporary deprivation, interspersed with binges and guilt.

Think of your mind as a computer. By daily reprogramming of your subconscious mind with healthy, positive data such as the affirmations on the next page, you can change your perspective toward eating. Your own mind can become a powerful aid in becoming your personal best.

As a yoga student, you spend time and effort on your body. You respect your body, your tool for life. Gradually, you will prefer the foods you deserve. As you replace a cup of coffee with juice, a donut with an apple, a soda with water and lemon, you will slowly feel better, gain pride and control, and look better. Then you will realize that the real food fadists are not the health-food nuts, but the people who are addicted to consuming junk food.

These yoga principles of eating provide a simple guide to good eating for better health and weight control. Your friends may notice changes in you and ask, "Are you on a diet?" Of course you are! Everyone is. We have come to use the word "diet" to mean a temporary food regime, but your yoga diet will become a way of life. And it will nurture you for a lifetime. Bon Appetit!

Mind-Set Strategy
for
Weight Loss

*I will respect my body and honor
it only with the food it deserves.*

*I will double my exercise and cut
my dietary intake in half until I reach
my ideal weight.*

*I will eat sparingly of the most
nutritious foods available. I will eat
something fresh and raw every day.*

*I will eat only when hungry . . .
never from boredom or loneliness.*

*I will replace the pleasure I seek
from food with constructive habits such
as listening to music, talking with a friend,
reading, taking a walk, or enjoying
a hobby.*

*I will not desire harmful foods. I
will see them as attractive robbers of
my potential personal best.*

*I am in control. I am becoming
the change I want to see happen.*

VII

The Yoga "I Can" Philosophy

The basic principles of yoga are: proper exercise, proper breathing, proper nutrition, proper relaxation, and proper thinking.

Of these, proper or positive thinking is probably the least emphasized. This path of yoga is a philosophy for control of mind and mastery of senses. Students learn that our moods don't dictate our thoughts—It's just the opposite: our thoughts, which we master, influence our moods. Therefore, "As I think, I am."

At first, it might seem that this "mental yoga" is contradictory, even incompatible, with Hatha Yoga's physical postures. Not so. In fact, the reverse is true: the hard work of physical discipline trains the mind, and the physical stretching creates a "flexibility" of the mind. Thus they compliment each other, forming a synergistic approach toward health. Just ask the student holding a pose—Hatha Yoga can be mind-bending!

No Judging No Grudging

Yoga philosophy encourages the student to judge neither himself nor others. We all know people who spend their lives striving to conform, to win approval, to do what is expected of them, and to fit into rigid standards of behavior that perpetuate this conformity. These standards bear rules for living that invariably contain words like *should, must, don't, can't,* and *always.* "Men *don't* cry," "Women *can't* act that way," "You *should* mop your floor every Friday," "Our family has *always* lived in this area." Yoga students learn to discard these external measures used to judge themselves and others. Each individual is unique with a private sense of purpose.

Many Gentle Yoga students come to class with judgments about their bodies which bewilder and confound them. We try to teach them that their bodies are not impediments but tools of attainment, to be appreciated and cherished.

Marvel at your body's design! A cut, an infection, a fracture, even abusive lifestyle habits, are testaments to the body's innate adaptive ability to heal itself, whether it gets medical treatment or not. If you eat something to which you are allergic, your body may exhibit a rash—the skin's way of eliminating toxins and warning you—and then clear up within a few hours. With inherent wisdom, and without rest, your body regulates a constantly changing internal environment. Respect your body and concentrate on its wonders rather than its short-comings. You may be amazed by your body's self-healing abilities.

Self-study enables the yoga student to deal with all the people and problems he encounters upon his path. If you blame your family, your doctor, your disease, or circum-stances for your unhappiness, you are at their mercy, thus making them responsible and you a helpless pawn. This sort of grudging keeps the focus off you, as well as the re-sponsibility. Negative thoughts such as "My husband makes me so mad" or "My disease makes it impossible for me to do that" turn you into a helpless victim. A truer assessment is to say, "I'm allowing my negative thoughts to control me." Remember: you are in charge of your own happiness, you are the master of your own situation, and don't surrender that right. No one, nothing, can take away your freedom to choose how you react.

Here we owe some space to your attitude toward your doctor. Ideally, s/he is a sensitive, up-to-date person who has treated you gently and fairly, but this is not always the case. Many students with chronic diseases harbor resent-ments toward doctors. Bear in mind that anger and denial are natural parts of your adjustment, necessary steps in the acceptance of your diagnosis in its proper perspective before you can get on with the living of life. But know that harboring deep-seated resentment toward your doctor may be unfair. Such resentment affects your mental health. Negative thoughts usually contain gross distortions and can color your moods with gloom and suffering. So, if you feel resentments of this kind, try to remember that every doctor is human and makes mistakes. If you have been unlucky, try to spend no more time on regret. Forgive. So much of our living is in the mind that we must monitor what we think.

Practice "Detachment"

Detachment is an ancient yogic technique. It is frequently misunderstood as disinterest or not caring. Actually it is a mind-set which allows the individual freedom to behave outside the binding forces of stress and emotion.

Envision yourself as swimming in a great ocean of life. By our actions, we set big waves into motion. And by the same big waves, we shall be hit *unless we learn to get out of the ocean.*

The following technique is helpful: Visualize yourself in a stressful situation. Then, as though you were being lifted up, observe the action as though from the ceiling of the room. Then observe yourself observing. Lift even higher, witnessing the players from a distant perspective in their relationship to the sun, the planet, the stars. Know that they are a small part of Nature's drama. This perspective is one of intuitive solidarity which allows fewer of those emotions which distort our thoughts and affect our body chemistry. With detachment, we can calm the ocean that surrounds our emotional body.

Re-Think Your Life In The Now

WE are the NOW generation. Yoga philosophy encourages you to give up the past in favor of the life you are living right now. Consider worry, regret, grudges, guilt, and anger as excess baggage and a needless waste of energy. If you reflect upon your life, you may be surprised by how much luggage you've been carrying around. Many middle-aged people still become embarrassed or humiliated just thinking about something that happened when they were teenagers! Initially, your conscience can point out errors, but once they are behind you, learn to drop them. Resolve to examine these past incidents from a detached perspective, and apply the Law of Karma: There is a reason for all things, a design to the occurrences in life, as there is a pattern to the Universe. Many of life's experiences which seem disastrous provide opportunities to learn the very lessons we need. Each of life's problems has a gift within it.

NOW is the only time you really ever have. In these pages, you have been reminded to "be aware," to become "detached," to "witness" what is happening to you. Few of us live in the present-moment awareness or even fully understand it. It is a state in which you do whatever you are doing with total wholeheartedness, without thinking of anything else, without hesitation, doubt, or inhibition of any kind. It is pure and timeless and totally absorbing. You may have experienced it while painting a picture, writing a poem, or listening to beautiful music. Little children play with NOW intensity. Realistically, we can't attain this awareness continually, but its memory can remind us to give up both the past and the future in favor of NOW life experience.

Make Things Happen

Open yourself up to new experiences. When a spontaneous invitation comes your way, do you automatically say "I can't" without having a good reason? Sometimes those unplanned experiences become precious memories, the unexpected opportunities, the turning points in our lives. Don't wait for the phone to ring. Be the initiator. Look for chances to extend your hospitality to others. Surround yourself with kindred spirits who share, support, and understand. Be the friend you would like to have yourself.

To gain perspective, think of your life as a drop in the millenium bucket. None of us has more. Use your time fully. How could you change your life for the better? Is there something you always meant to do? Act out a fantasy! Take that trip! Send those flowers! Today is all any of us has. When it's all said and done, which epitaph would you rather have? "She kept her house clean," "He did his duty," or "She taught me to laugh," "He was a wonderful friend." Re-think your life regularly and reevaluate your priorities.

See yourself as free of boundaries, growth-oriented, ever-learning—moving toward a limitless potential.

*It is never
how high one rises
that determines one's merit,
but rather
how far one has come,
considering his
difficulties.*

—*Archibald Rutledge*

VIII

Meet Our Models

Hoping that they will inspire you as they have inspired us, we want you to meet six members of our Gentle Yoga class at the YWCA in Cedar Rapids, Iowa.

Our class meets once a week for two hours. We begin class together with yoga breathing, neck rolls, and eye exercises. Then each student continues with an individualized list of postures to practice. The class ends with relaxation.

The students in our Gentle Yoga class are devoted to yoga. Most of them have also been treated or are under treatment by a physical therapy department, but they are amazed that something which seems as simple as yoga can make such appreciable differences in their symptoms and overall health. We believe this is due in part to yoga's basic concept of self-responsibility. The students have the courage to cope with their physical limitations with perseverance and to focus on what they *can* do rather than on what they *can't* do. They leave class invigorated, relaxed, smiling, and pleased with themselves and their progress.

They are very special people.

Cleatus Creel

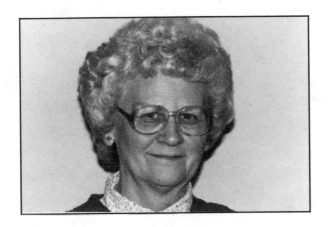

Cleatus Creel is a warm cheerful person with a peaches-and-cream complexion, beautiful pure white hair, and a determination to retain her flexibility despite arthritis. After her three sons were grown, Cleatus returned to work as a medical secretary and receptionist and continued working until recently. She loves gardening—and her baby grandson who lives nearby is her delight.

Arthritis struck Cleatus in 1981. It began with sore wrists, then moved rapidly to other joints. When she began doing yoga, her shoulders were extremely tight, but in only two months, she increased her shoulder flexibility by five inches. (See page 90.) Although she experiences good and bad days, she is getting along well with lots of rest, aspirin, and yoga.

"I can't say enough good things about yoga," Cleatus says. "I highly recommend it to anyone with mobility problems due to arthritis. It keeps you moving."

Tom Eisen

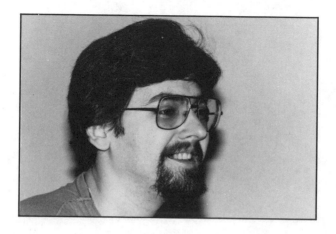

Born in Kansas City and a graduate of the University of Missouri's School of Journalism, Tom Eisen is a friendly, out-going 29-year-old television reporter who specializes in consumer affairs. His bouts of dizziness, blurred vision, and extreme fatigue were diagnosed as multiple sclerosis a month before his 26th birthday. Typical of his sensitive desire to reach out to others, Tom soon started an M.S. support group where information and common concerns are shared at monthly meetings.

"Most of my battle has been fighting fatigue," says Tom. "An M.S. patient wakes up with a daily allotment of energy; you must ration it prudently so that you don't run out before evening." He also warns M.S. patients not to read any information about multiple sclerosis which is more than five years old because old concepts are discouraging. New statistics reveal that 75% of victims are still not disabled twenty years after their diagnosis.

Arlene Henderson

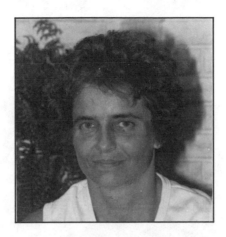

Arlene Henderson is 43 years old, the mother of two children, and the proud grandmother of a new granddaughter. Although she is confined to a wheelchair, she lives alone in her own home. Twice a week, a visiting homemaker helps her with washing, cleaning and similar odd jobs, and Arlene is determined to continue to live independently. By using the local bus for the handicapped, she manages to do her own grocery shopping and to come to the YWCA for our weekly yoga classes.

Arlene was only 18 and had just graduated from high school when she suffered her first attack of M.S. The disease was diagnosed a year later. She is an enthusiastic yoga student and never misses a class. She says yoga makes her feel alive and not just part of a wheelchair. We lift her onto a floor mat where she is able to do many postures including a fabulous forward bend. Her favorite posture is shoulder stand which we help her with at the end of each class.

Arlene's cheerful determination inspires all of us.

Lucy Hinz

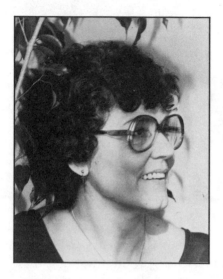

Lucy Hinz is tall, dark-haired, attractive, and looks years younger than her age of 51. She is married to "a wonderful supportive husband," is the mother of three grown daughters, and has one grandson. Her special joys are bridge and golf.

Although doctors say her M.S. was probably coming on for ten years, it was finally diagnosed six years ago when she suffered an acute onset of aching, double vision, numbness and shaking. For three months, she was in a wheelchair. Then gradually, she improved enough to walk with a walker, then with a cane, and she now walks unassisted. Each step of her improvement was a triumph and the result of determination, optimism and hard work.

Lucy's advice to others: "Don't ever give up. There's always a tomorrow which can turn out to be wonderful."

John Jenney

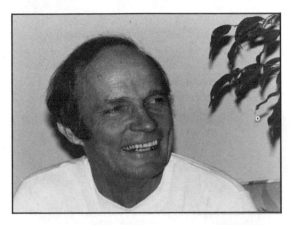

John Jenney has a twinkle in his eye and a smile that is habitual. He was born in 1929 and was a pilot in the Korean War. John is married and is the father of six children between the ages of 17 and 25. For years he was a wholesale distributor of floor coverings and travelled throughout Iowa. He was well-known locally as an outstanding golfer.

John's M.S. symptoms appeared gradually. Looking back, he can remember tell-tale signs, but they didn't last and didn't seem worth investigating. However, in September 1976, John developed a serious limp which didn't go away. In May of 1977, the final diagnosis was made: multiple sclerosis.

John is enthusiastic about yoga. "Our two hour yoga class and the relaxation period and positive attitude have helped me considerably. My balance has definitely improved, and many of the postures use muscles that are stimulated by nerves I haven't used due to the spasticity of my left side."

His advice to other MSers: "Don't quit. Take advantage of every program offered and keep using and improving your body. You can't give up."

Marilyn Sand

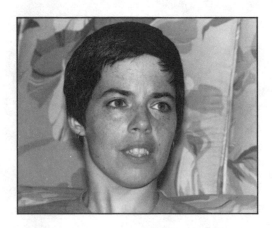

Marilyn Sand's warm smile and pixie-like appearance endear her to everyone who meets her. She is 29, married, the mother of a two-year-old daughter who looks just like her—and she has rheumatoid arthritis.

Marilyn was a high school science teacher in 1977 when her first symptoms appeared. Beginning in the joints of her fingers, the swelling and pain later spread to all the joints of her body. She is especially grateful for the support of her husband: "We'd only been married two years when I developed arthritis so my husband faced the in-sickness-in-health test early."

Marilyn's major problems are painful shoulders and knees, and tight hip joints. She especially enjoys the chest expander, bridge, and shoulder stand against a wall.

Her advice: "I think it's essential to find the right doctor. Look for a specialist who understands arthritis and who will treat you intelligently."

Suggested Reading List

If you wish to learn more about the various subjects discussed in this book, the following titles are recommended. These are just a sampling. Many excellent books have been omitted.

Bodywork

Carr, Rachel *ARTHRITIS: RELIEF BEYOND DRUGS*. New York, NY: Harper and Row, 1981

Christensen, A. and Rankin, D. *EASY DOES IT YOGA FOR OLDER PEOPLE*. New York, NY: Harper and Row, 1975

Couch, Jean and Weaver, Nell *RUNNER'S WORLD YOGA BOOK*. Mountain View, CA.: World Publications, 1979

Devi, Indra *FOREVER YOUNG, FOREVER HEALTHY*. New York, NY: Arco Publishing Company, 1975

Dychtwald, Ken *BODYMIND*. New York, NY: Jove Publications, 1978

Folan, Lilias *LILIAS, YOGA, AND YOUR LIFE*. New York, NY: Macmillan Publishing Co., 1981

Funderburk, James Ph.D. *SCIENCE STUDIES YOGA*. Honesdale, PA: Himalayan International Institute, 1977

Hittleman, Richard *YOGA 28 DAY EXERCISE PLAN*. New York, NY: Workman Publishing Co., 1969

Iyengar, B.K.S. *LIGHT ON YOGA*. New York, NY: Schocken Books: 1965

Kraus, Hans, M.D. *BACKACHE, STRESS AND TENSION*. New York, NY: Simon and Schuster, 1965

Norton, Suza *YOGA FOR PEOPLE OVER FIFTY*. Old Greenwich, CT: Devin-Adair, 1977

Swami Vishnu Devananda *THE COMPLETE ILLUSTRATED BOOK OF YOGA*. New York, NY: Bell Publishing Co. Inc., 1960

For Eyes

Bates, William, M.D. *BETTER EYESIGHT WITHOUT GLASSES*. New York, NY: Pyramid Books, 1940

The Healthy Mind

Benson, Herbert *THE RELAXATION RESPONSE.* New York, NY: William Morrow and Co., 1975

Bry A. with Bair, M. *DIRECTING THE MOVIES OF YOUR MIND.* New York, NY: Harper and Row, 1978

Cousins, Norman *ANATOMY OF AN ILLNESS.* New York, NY: W.W. Norton and Co., 1979

Cousins, Norman *HUMAN OPTIONS.* New York, NY: W.W. Norton and Co., 1981

Dyer, Wayne *YOUR ERRONEOUS ZONES.* New York, NY: Avon Books, 1976

Pelletier, Ken *MIND AS HEALER, MIND AS SLAYER.* New York, NY: Delacorte, 1977

Samuels, M. and Samuels, N. *SEEING WITH THE MIND'S EYE.* New York, NY: Random House, 1975

Simonton, Carl, Mathews-Simonton, Stephanie and Creighton, James *GETTING WELL AGAIN.* Los Angeles, CA. J.P. Tarcher, Inc., 1978

Nutrition

Ballantine, Rudolph, M.D. *DIET AND NUTRITION, A HOLISTIC APPROACH.* Honesdale, AP: Himalayan International Institute, 1978

Brody, Jane *JANE BRODY'S NUTRITION BOOK.* New York, NY: W.W. Norton and Co., 1981

Dufty, William *SUGAR BLUES.* New York, NY: Warner Books, 1976

Ewald, Ellen *RECIPES FOR A SMALL PLANET.* New York, NY: Ballantine Books, 1973

Hewitt, Jean *THE NEW YORK TIMES NATURAL FOODS COOKBOOK.* New York, NY: Avon Books, 1972

Lappe, Francis Moore *DIET FOR A SMALL PLANET.* New York, NY: Ballantine Books, 1977

Nurtition Search, Inc. John Kirshman, Director *NUTRITION ALMANAC.* New York, NY: McGraw Hill, 1973

Wright, Jonathan V. *DR. WRIGHT'S BOOK OF NUTRITIONAL THERAPY.* Emmaus, PA: Rodale Books, 1979

Wellness In General

Bach, Marcus *THE POWER OF TOTAL LIVING.* New York, NY: Dodd, Mead, and Co., 1977

Ferguson, Tom *MEDICAL SELF-CARE.* New York, NY: Summit Books, 1980

McCamy, John and Presley, James *HUMAN LIFESTYLING.* New York, NY: Harper and Row, 1975

Ryan, Regina Sara and Travis, John W. *THE WELLNESS WORKBOOK,* Berkeley, CA: Ten Speed Press, 1981

Multiple Sclerosis

Ottenberg, Miriam *THE PURSUIT OF HOPE.* New York, NY: Rawson, Wade Publishers, 1978

Magazines

AMERICAN HEALTH, Fitness of Body and Mind, Des Moines, IA.

PREVENTION, The Magazine for Better Health, Emmaus, PA

YOGA JOURNAL, California Yoga Teachers Association, Berkeley, CA

ACCENT ON LIVING, For the Physically Disabled, Bloomington, IL.

Supplement for Teachers

We are very pleased that so many teachers have formed classes for "gentle" people, and are using our book, GENTLE YOGA. When we wrote the book, our major focus was directed toward the individual student. However, we have since received many inquiries from teachers to whom we would like to pass along a few suggestions which we have developed by trial and error.

We suggest that you use a form such as our "Get Acquainted" form. This will establish a file on students, as well as help you remember details.

A second form, a composite of the poses, enables the teacher to circle appropriate poses for each student. We fill out two copies: one to be taken home, one to keep on file to refresh our memories.

Avail yourself of a current medical textbook and a medication reference such as THE PHYSICIAN'S DESK REFERENCE. A basic understanding of the various diseases is necessary; knowledge of students' medications and side effects will give you insight into why they fall asleep, have halitosis, suffer spasms, experience disposition changes.

Obtain prudent liability insurance. Then, with care, encourage wheelchair-bound students to sit on the floor. Prop them against the wall or a helper's back, but get them out of their chairs if possible! The wheelchair not only limits movement, but engenders a negative self-image and a psychological attachment.

Lastly, a strong, compassionate assistant is invaluable. If she has a yoga or medical background, you are truly fortunate. Knowledge of body mechanics and lifting techniques are also helpful.

Working with Gentle Yoga has been a very satisfying experience. May your work bring you joy. Please drop us a note and tell us what works for you.

Gentle Yoga "Get Acquainted" Form

Name

Address

Phone Number

Age

Special health problems:

Have you ever had high blood pressure?

Do you have thyroid problems or diabetes?

Are you taking any medication regularly? (The stimulus your endocrine system receives during the inverted positions may require a decreased dosage of some medications.)

Have you had recent surgery?

Do you use an I.U.D.? (If so, it's important to be careful with abdominal lifts. If you are going to lose an I.U.D., yoga will speed up the process.)

What do you hope to gain from taking yoga?

Please feel free to call me about any yoga-related problems you might have.

Teacher _____

Phone _____

Gentle Yoga

NAME_____

SPECIAL PROBLEMS_____

BREATHING

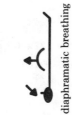 diaphramatic breathing   bellows breath   alternate nostril breath

NECK AND SHOULDERS

neck rolls   chest expander   rope stretches   warrior

FORWARD BENDING

TWIST

knees to side   T-twist

LATERAL BENDING

Atlas   grape picking   triangle II

HIP/THIGH JOINT

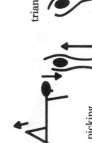
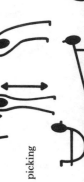

142

BACKWARD BENDING

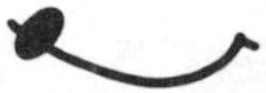

boat

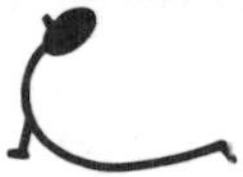

cobra

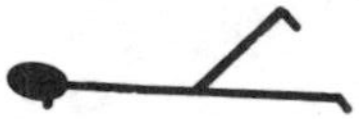

locust

forward bend

LEG STRETCHES

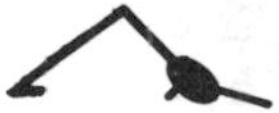

dog

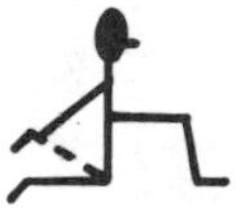

lunge

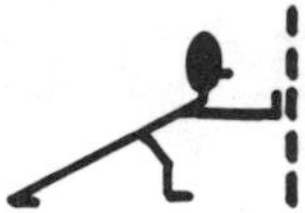

calf stretch

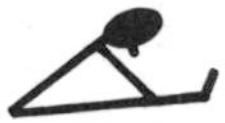

ceiling walk

ABDOMINAL TONERS

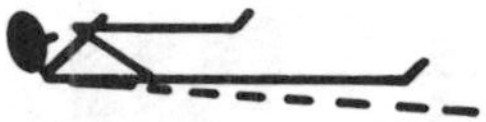

knee hug

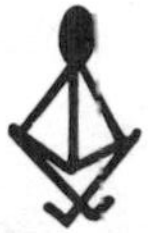

abdominal lift

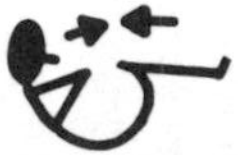

crunch

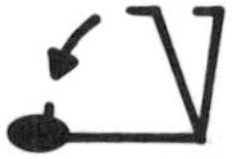

FINGERS AND HANDS

finger lift

hand warmer

REVERSE POSTURES

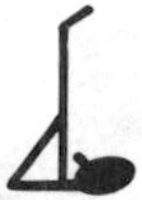

shoulder stand

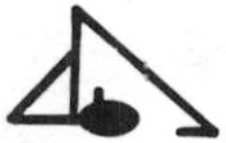

plough

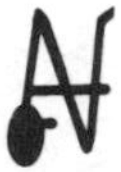

baby headstand

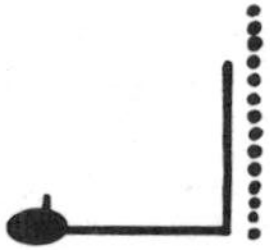

stick pose

EYE EXERCISES

RELAXATION

143

Other Books You May Enjoy...